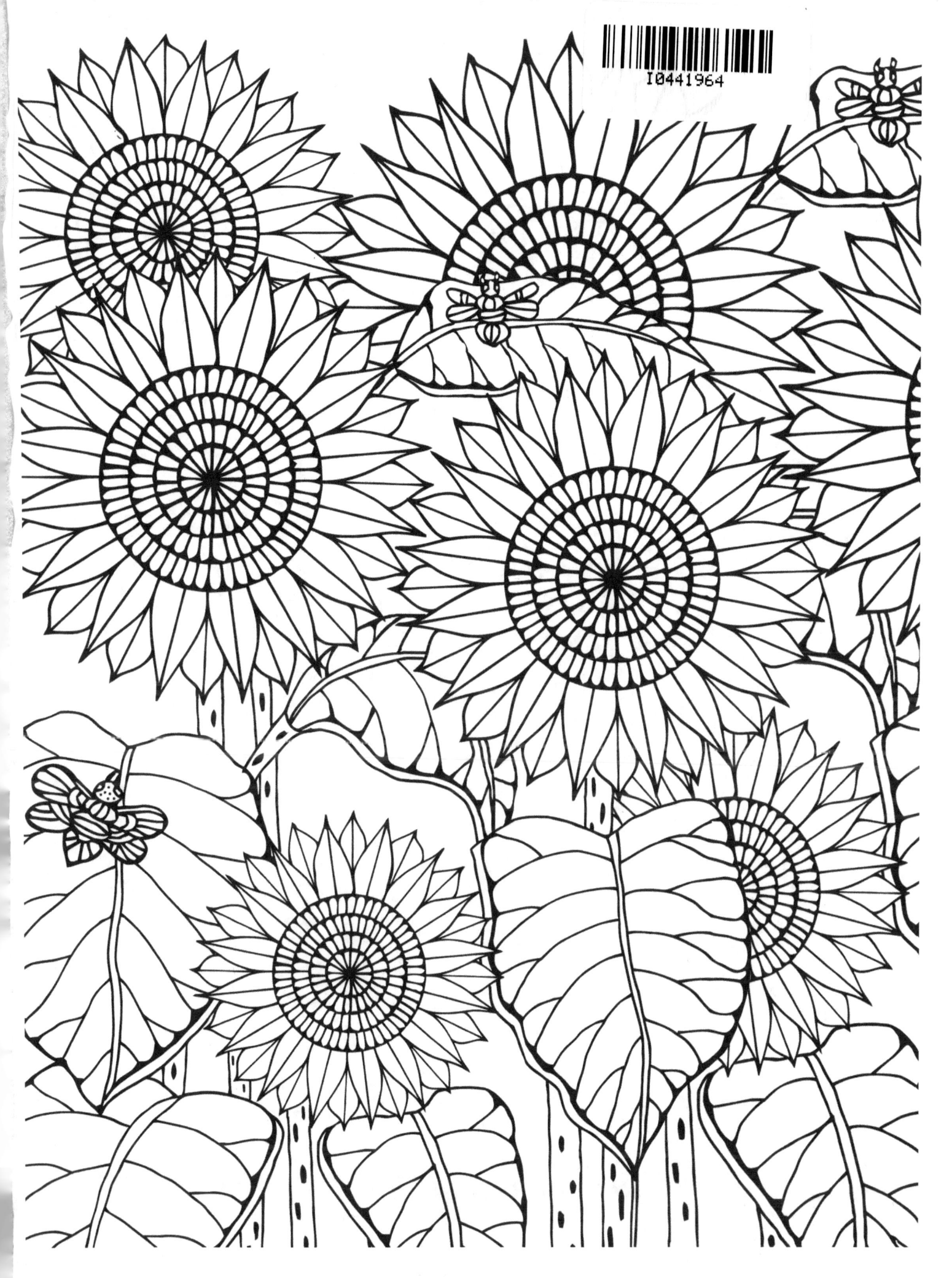

I0441964

Left blank for your convenience

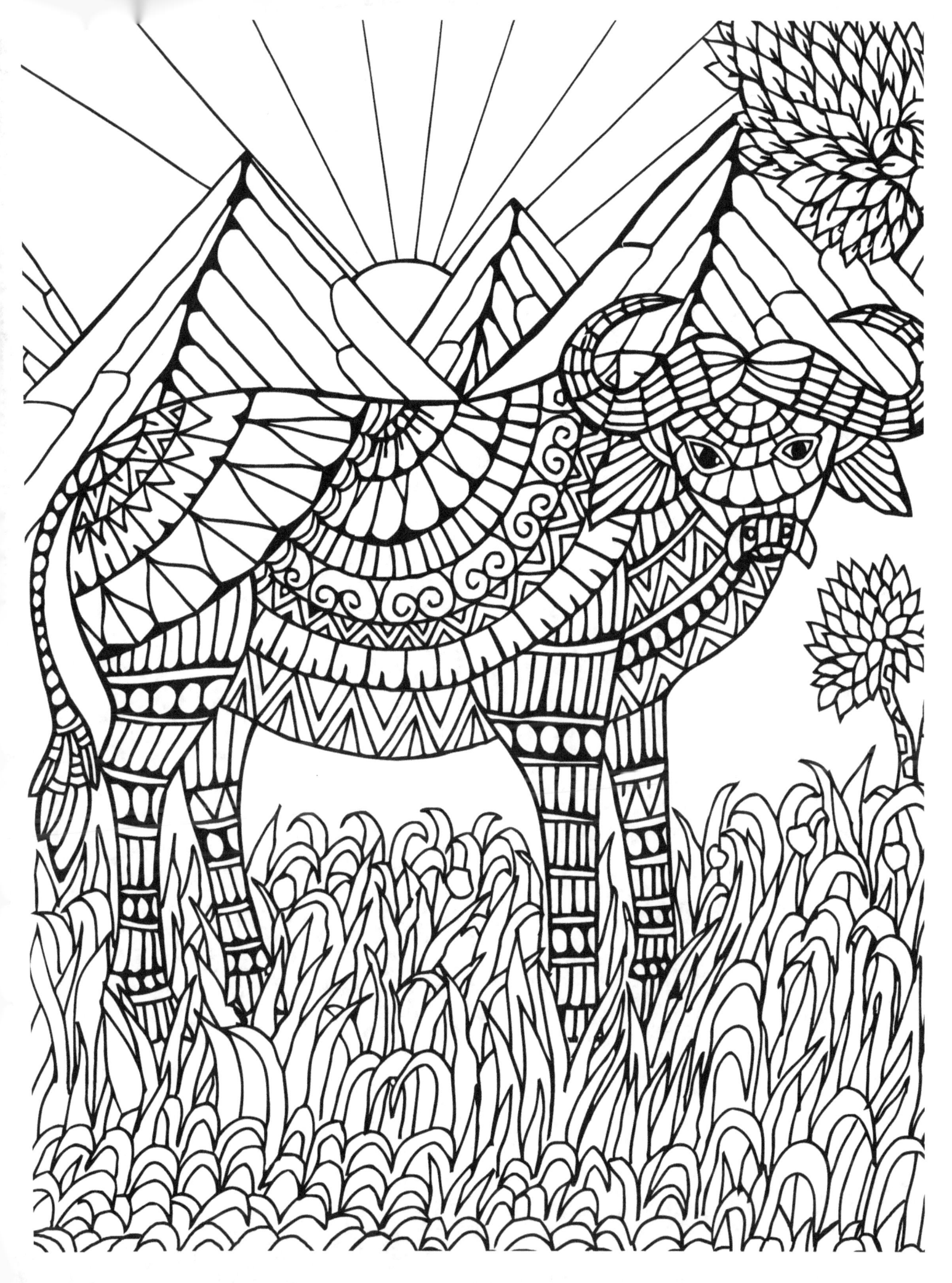

Left blank for your convenience

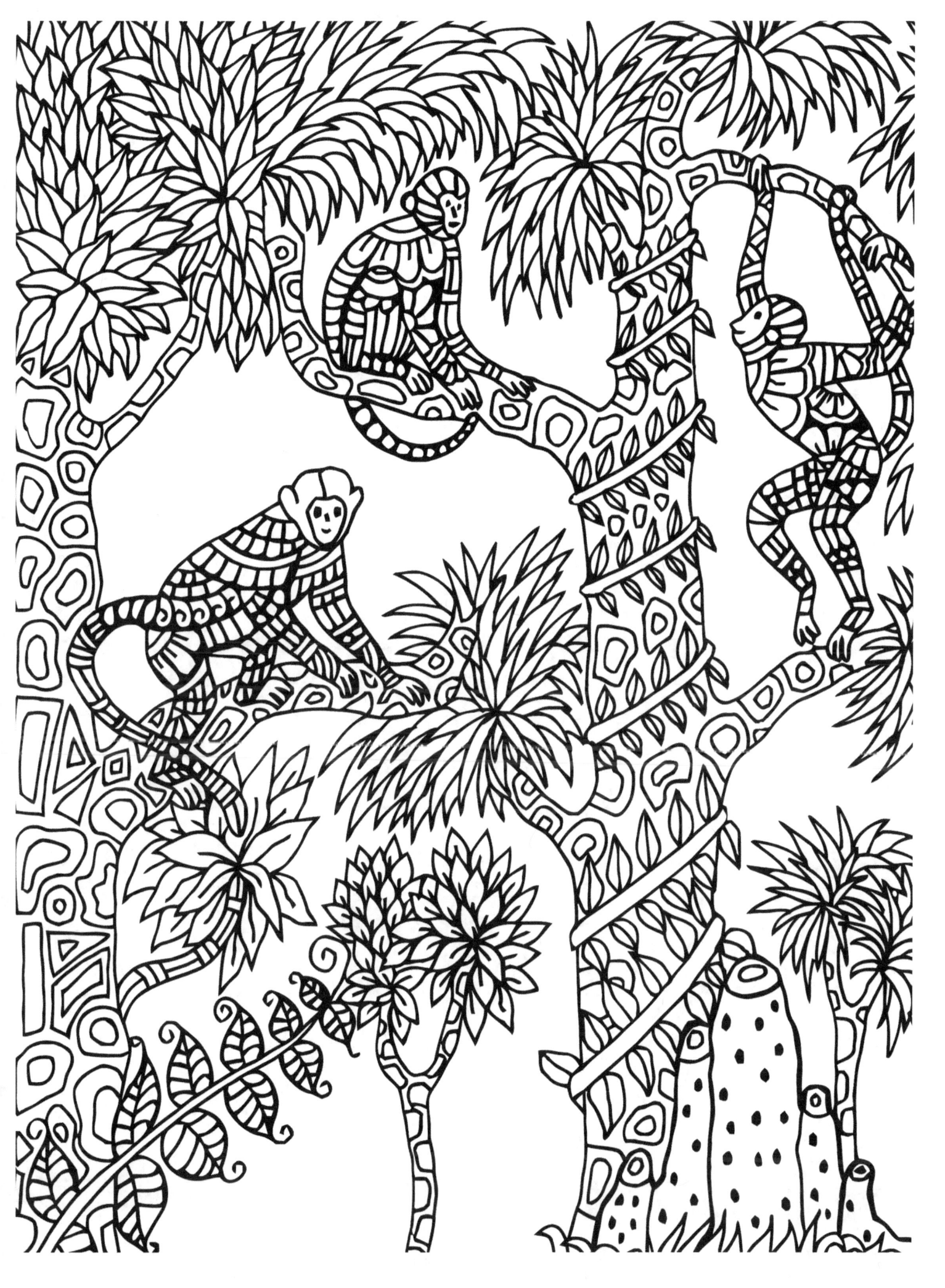

Left blank for your convenience

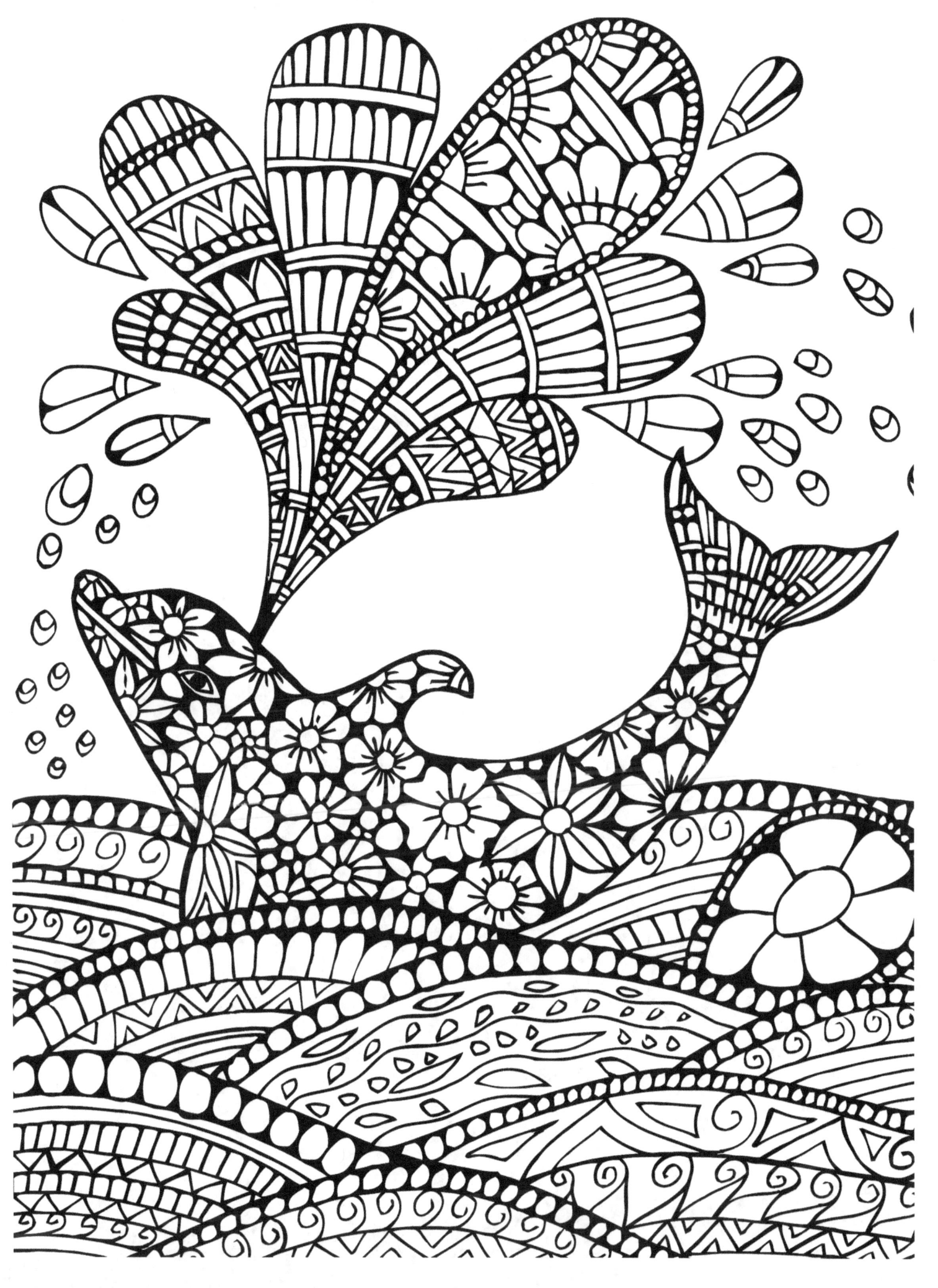

Left blank for your convenience

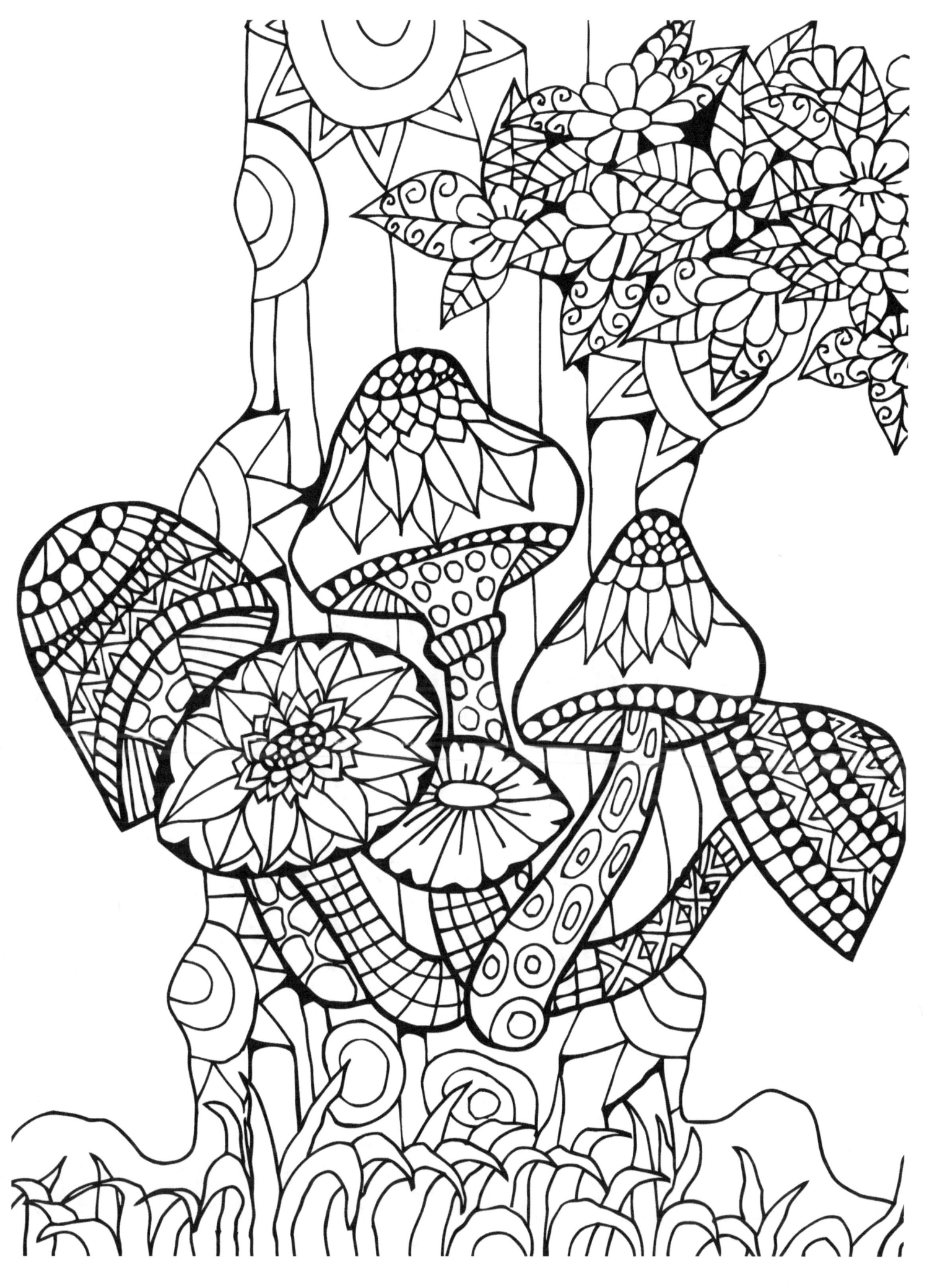

Left blank for your convenience

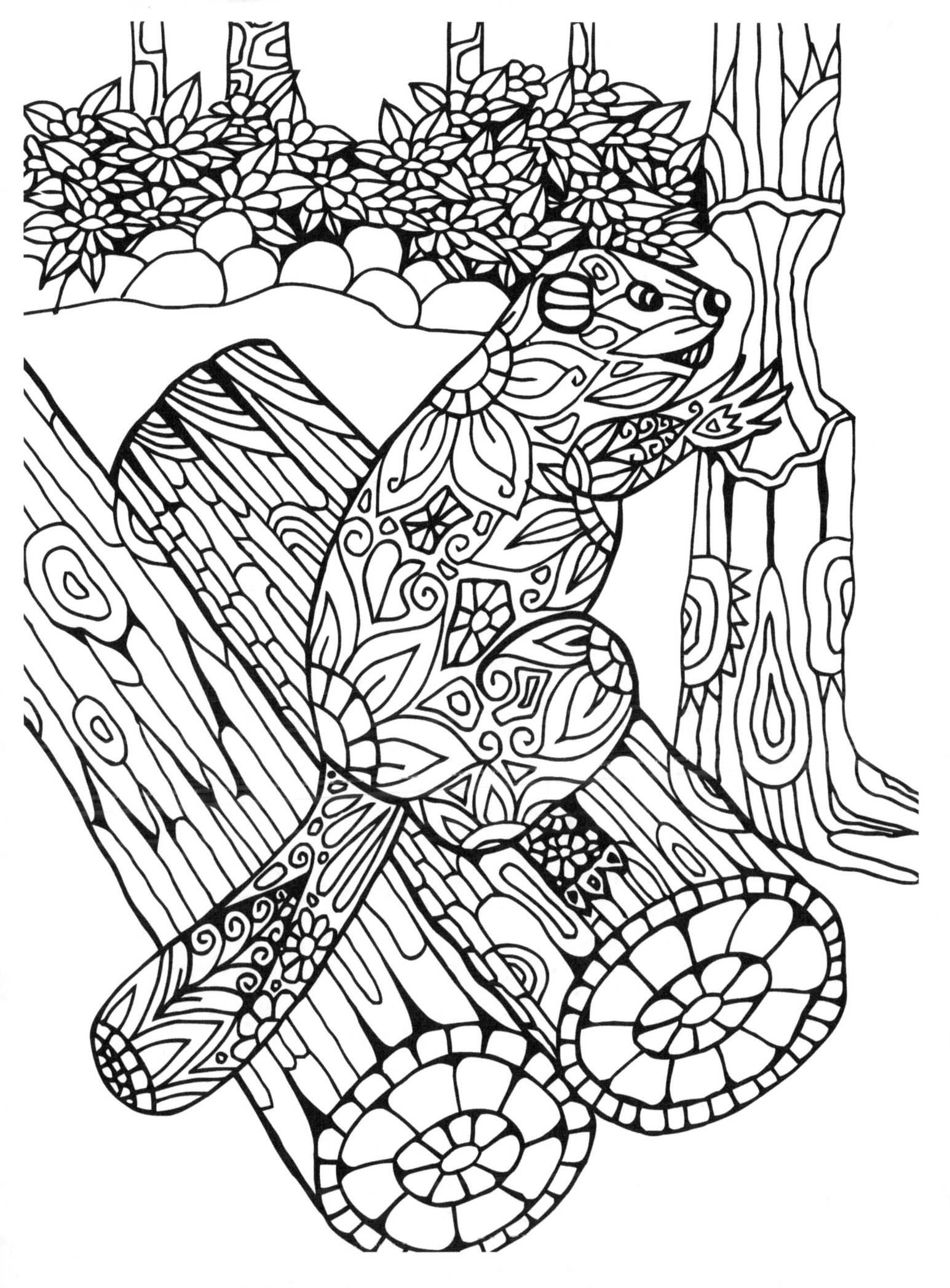

Left blank for your convenience

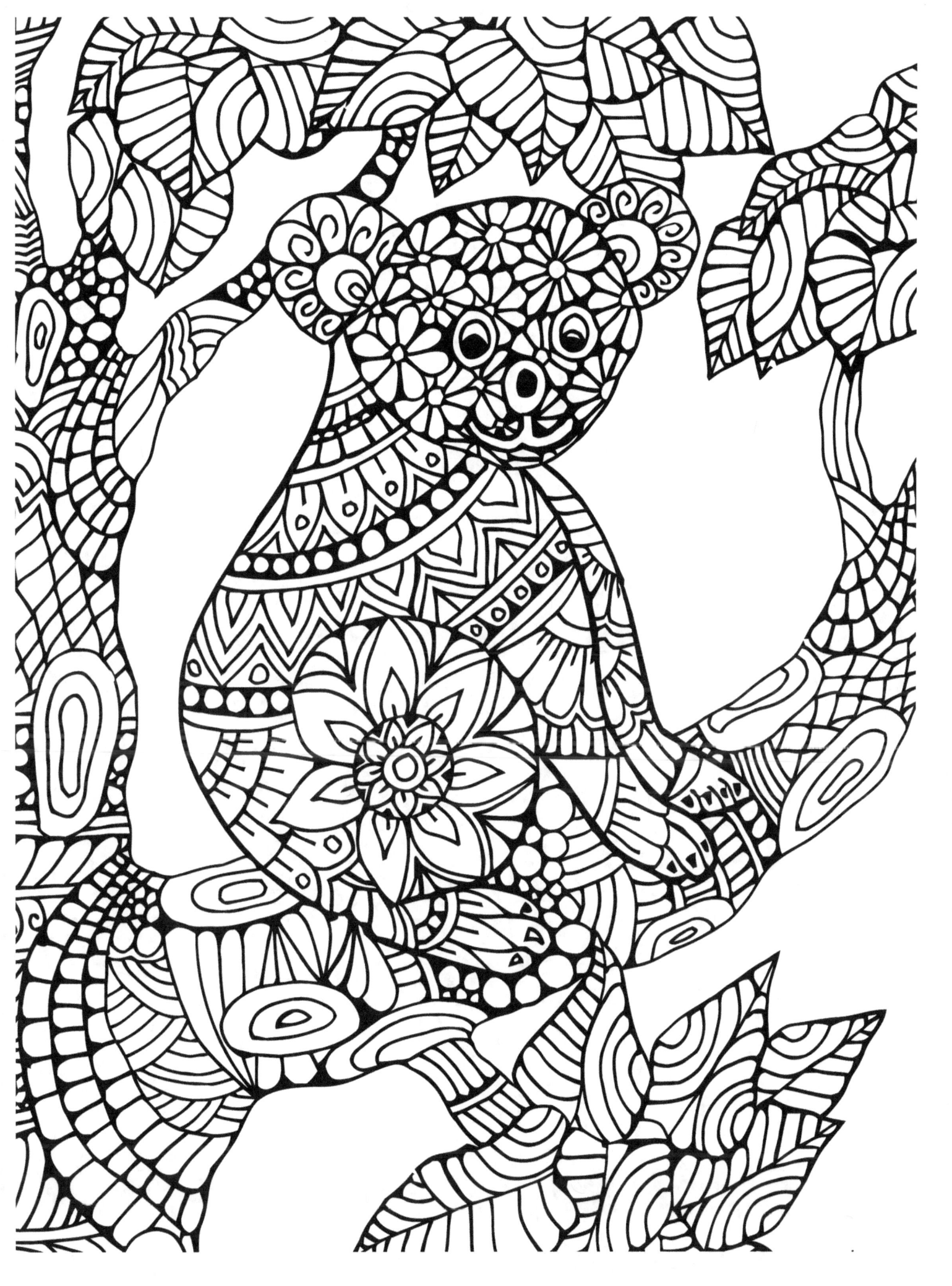

Left blank for your convenience

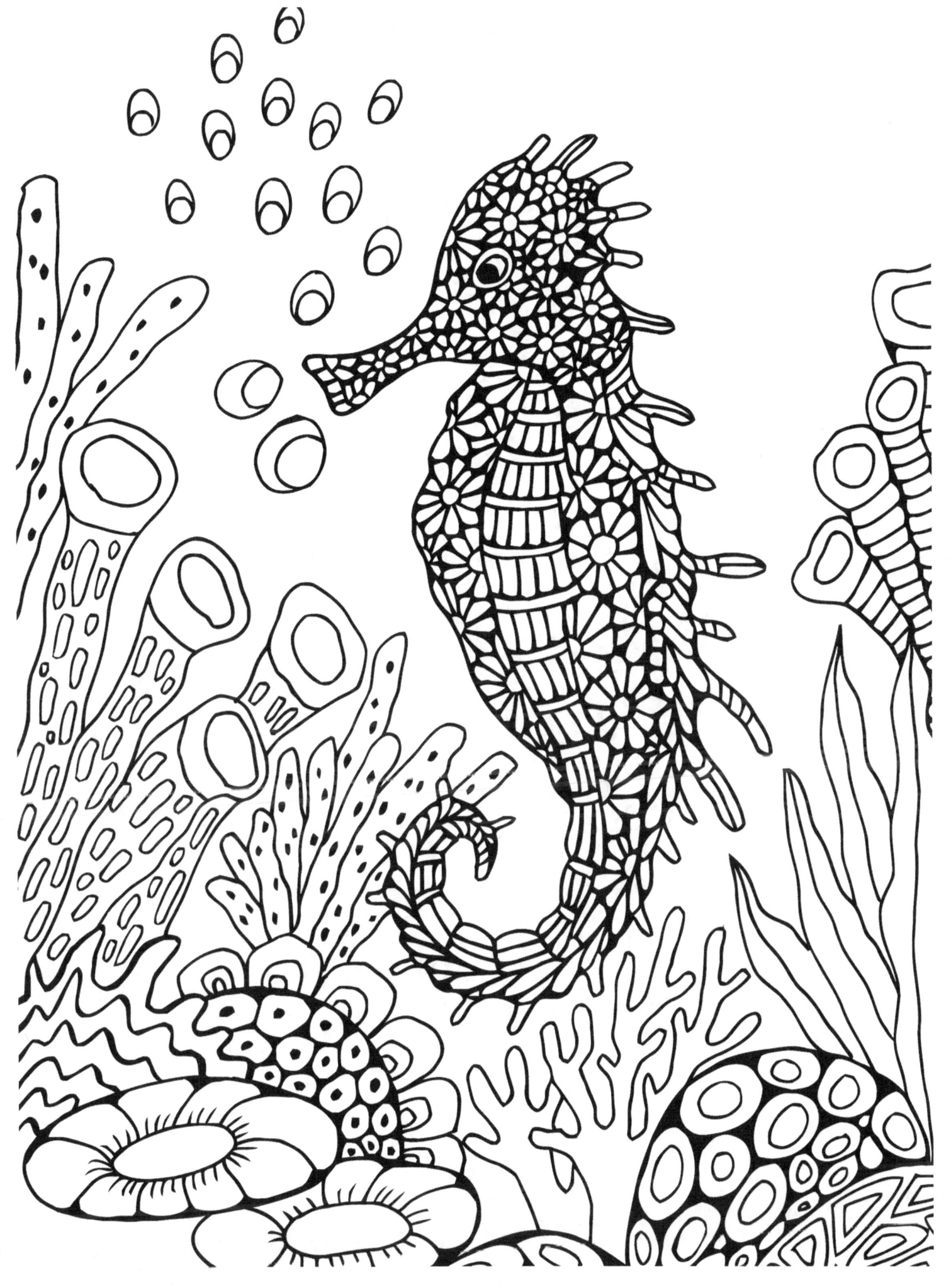

Left blank for your convenience

Left blank for your convenience

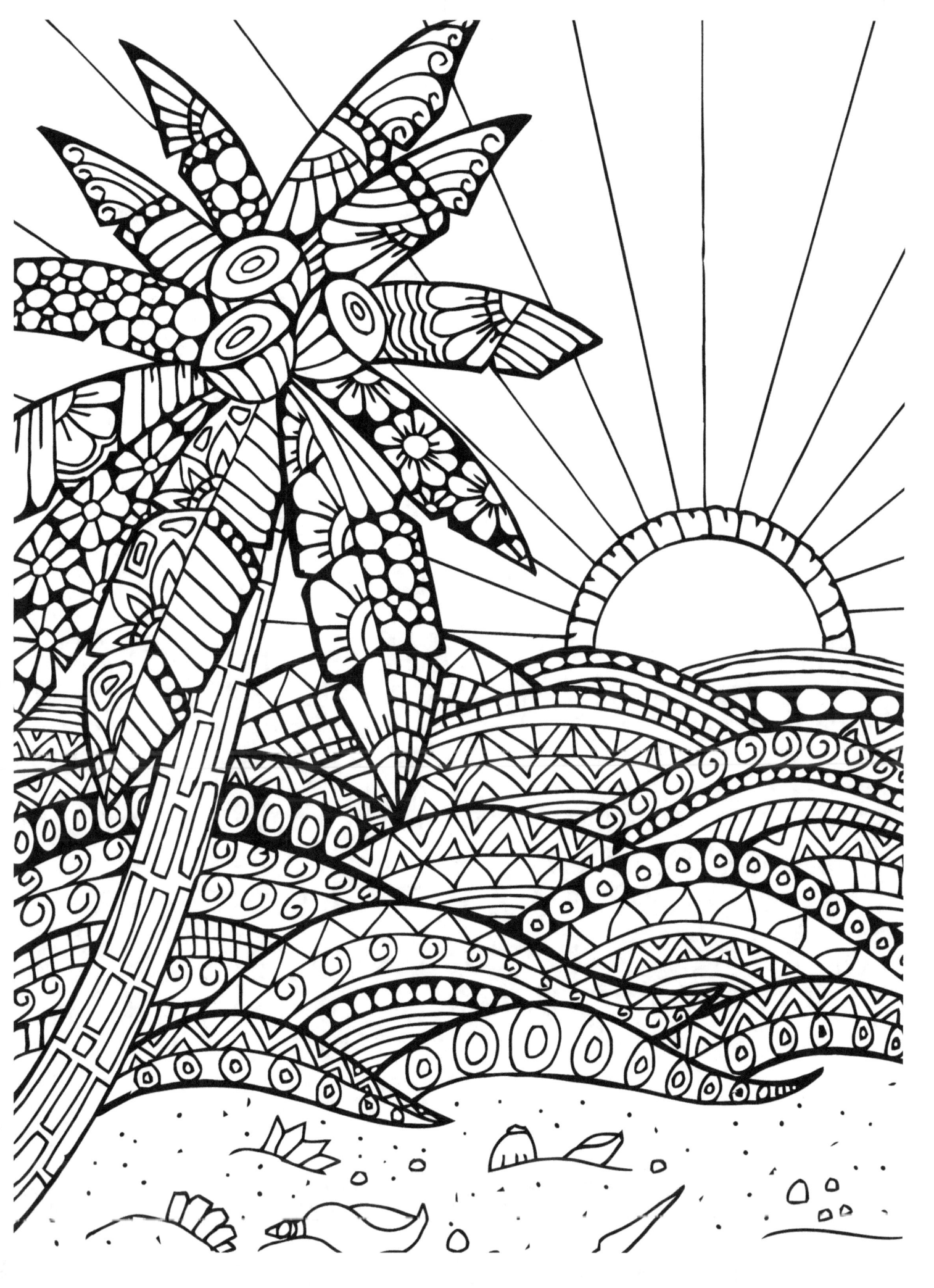

Left blank for your convenience

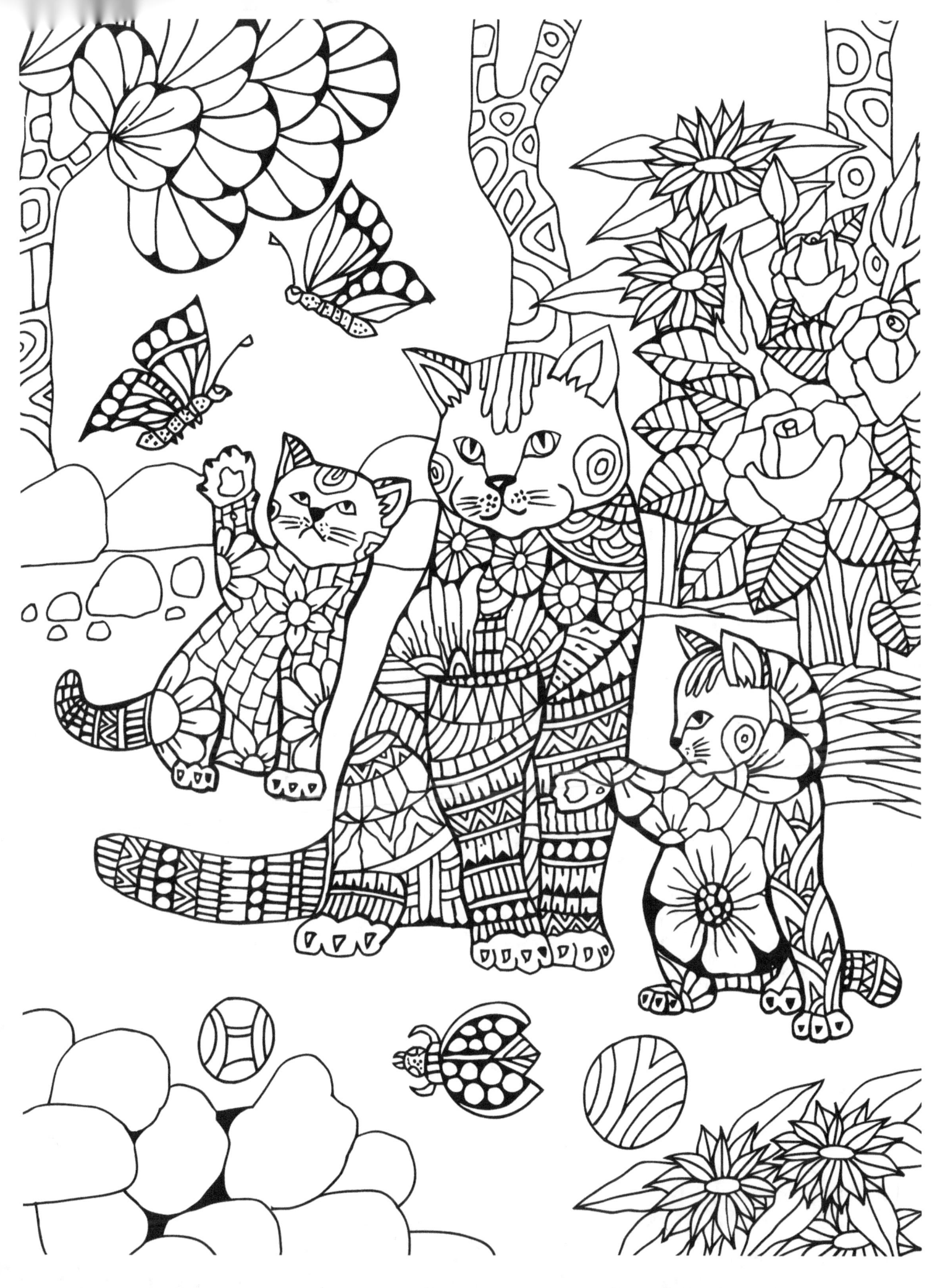

Left blank for your convenience

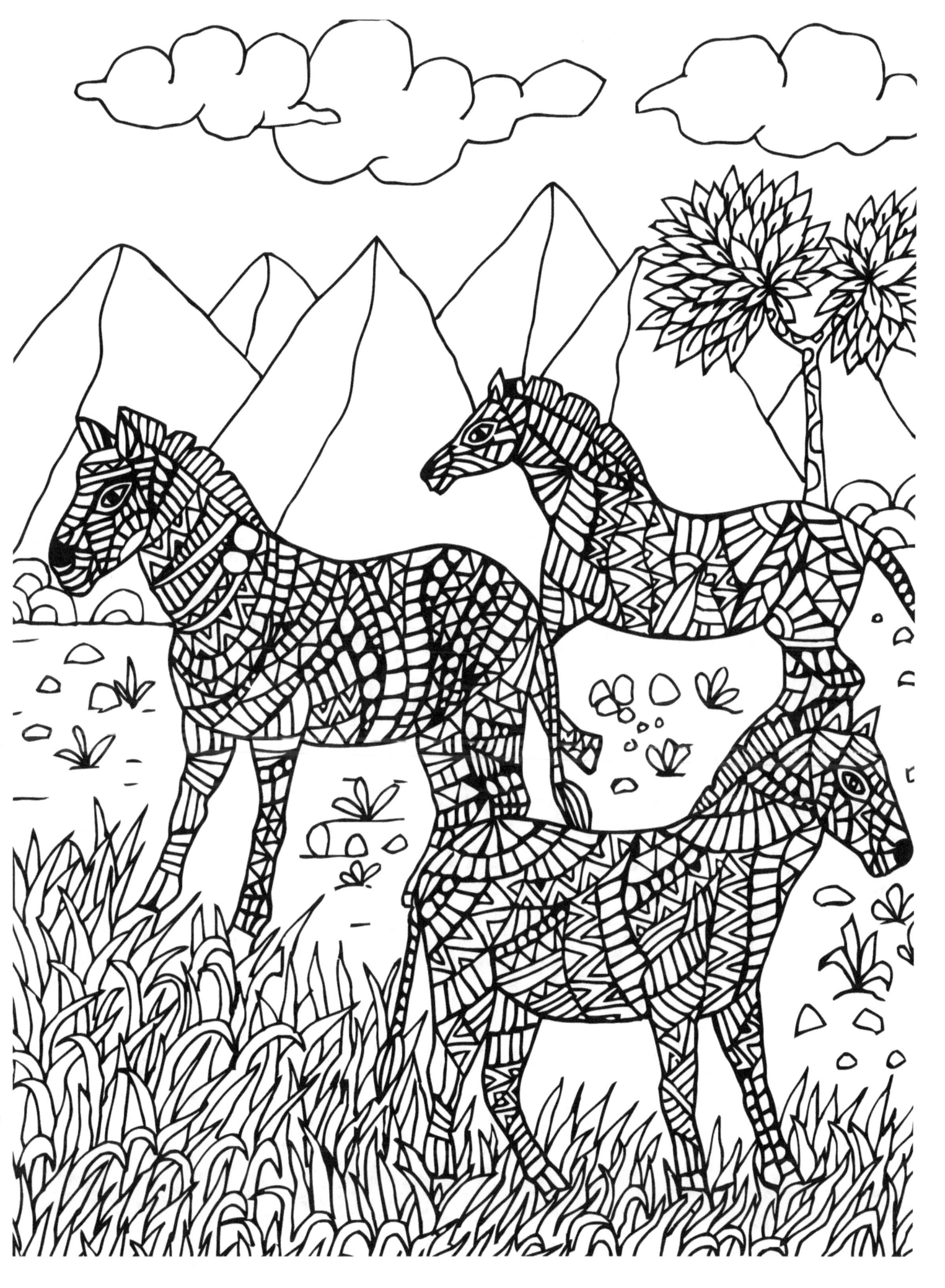

Left blank for your convenience

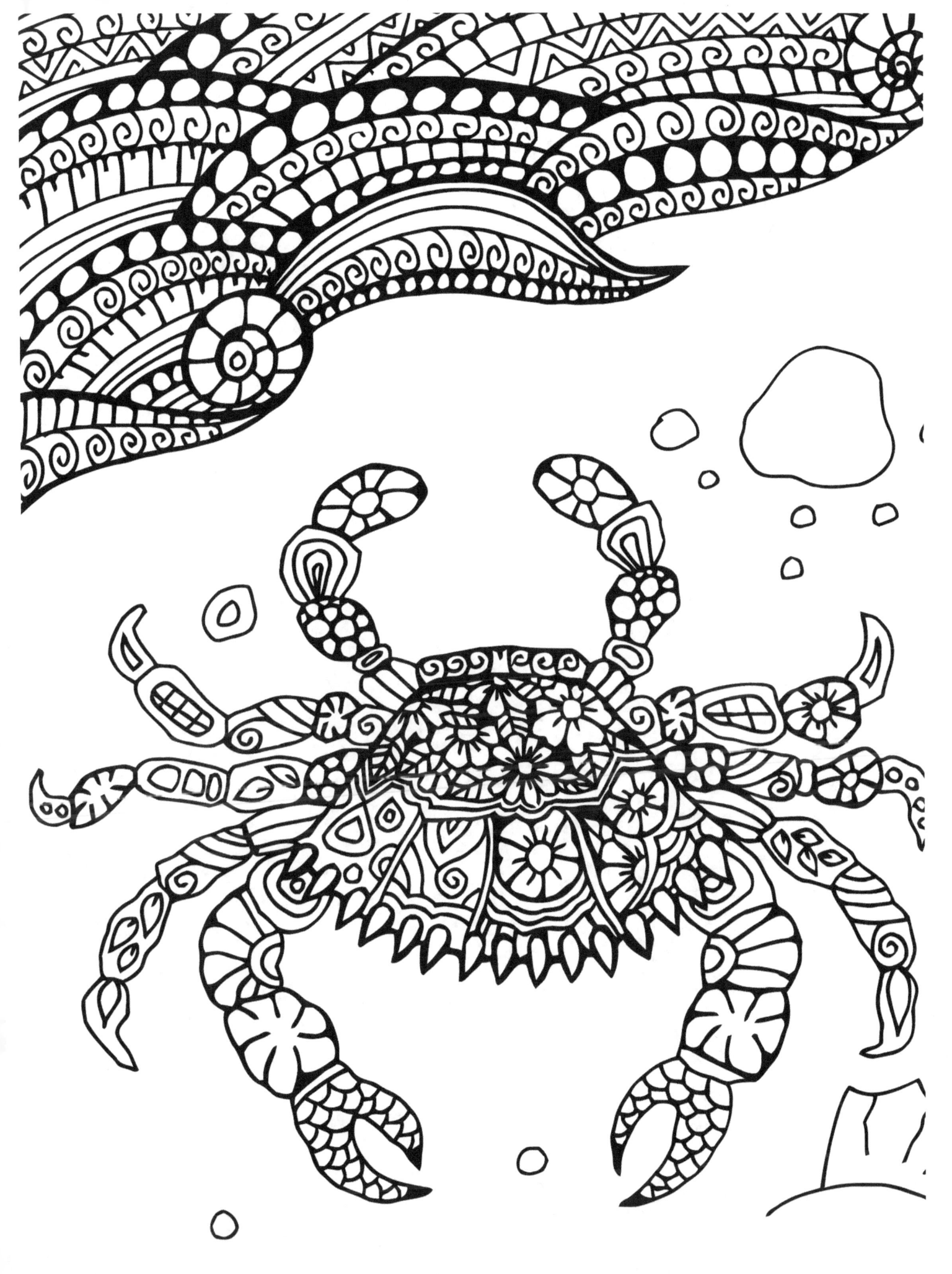

Left blank for your convenience

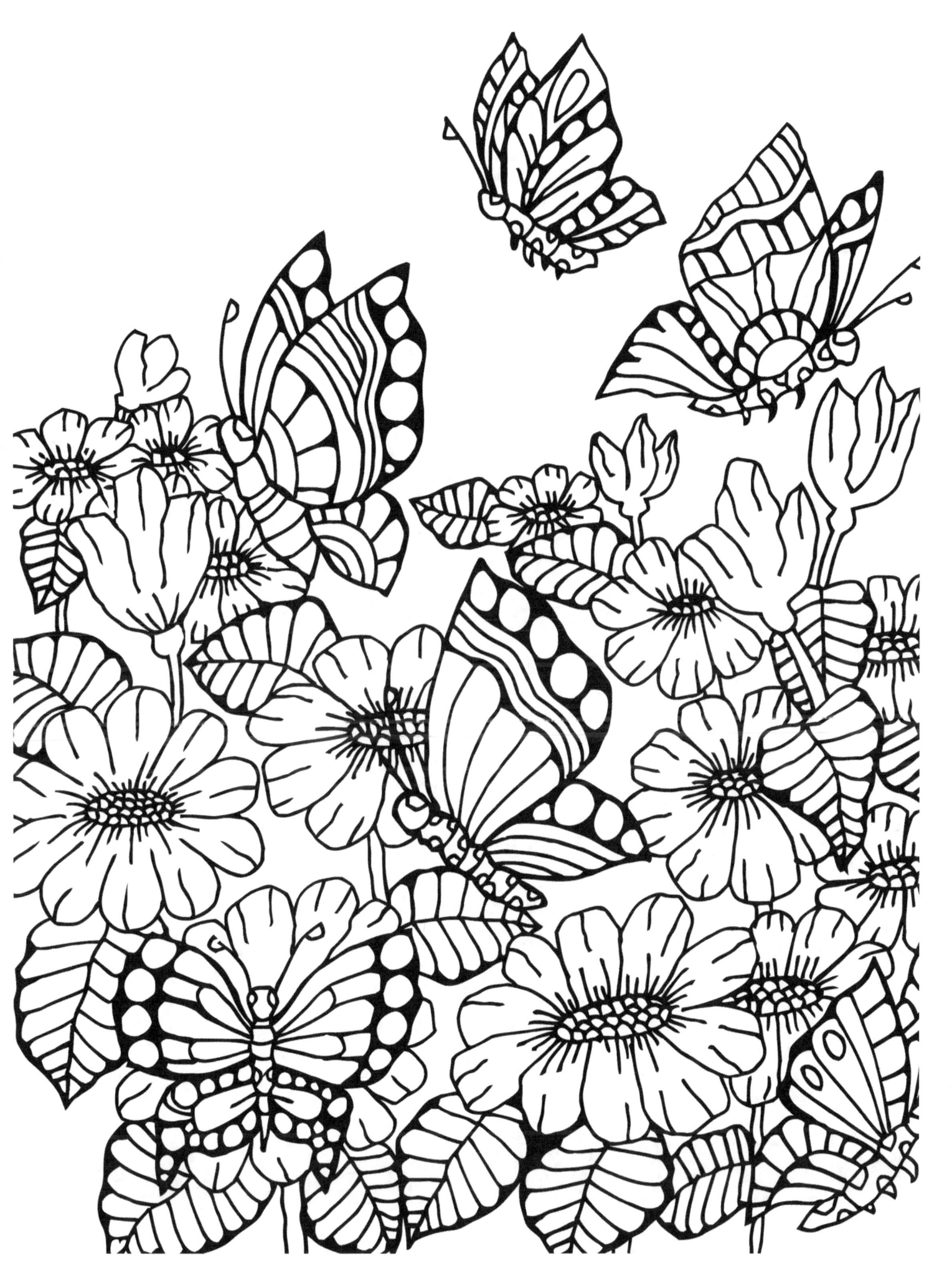

Left blank for your convenience

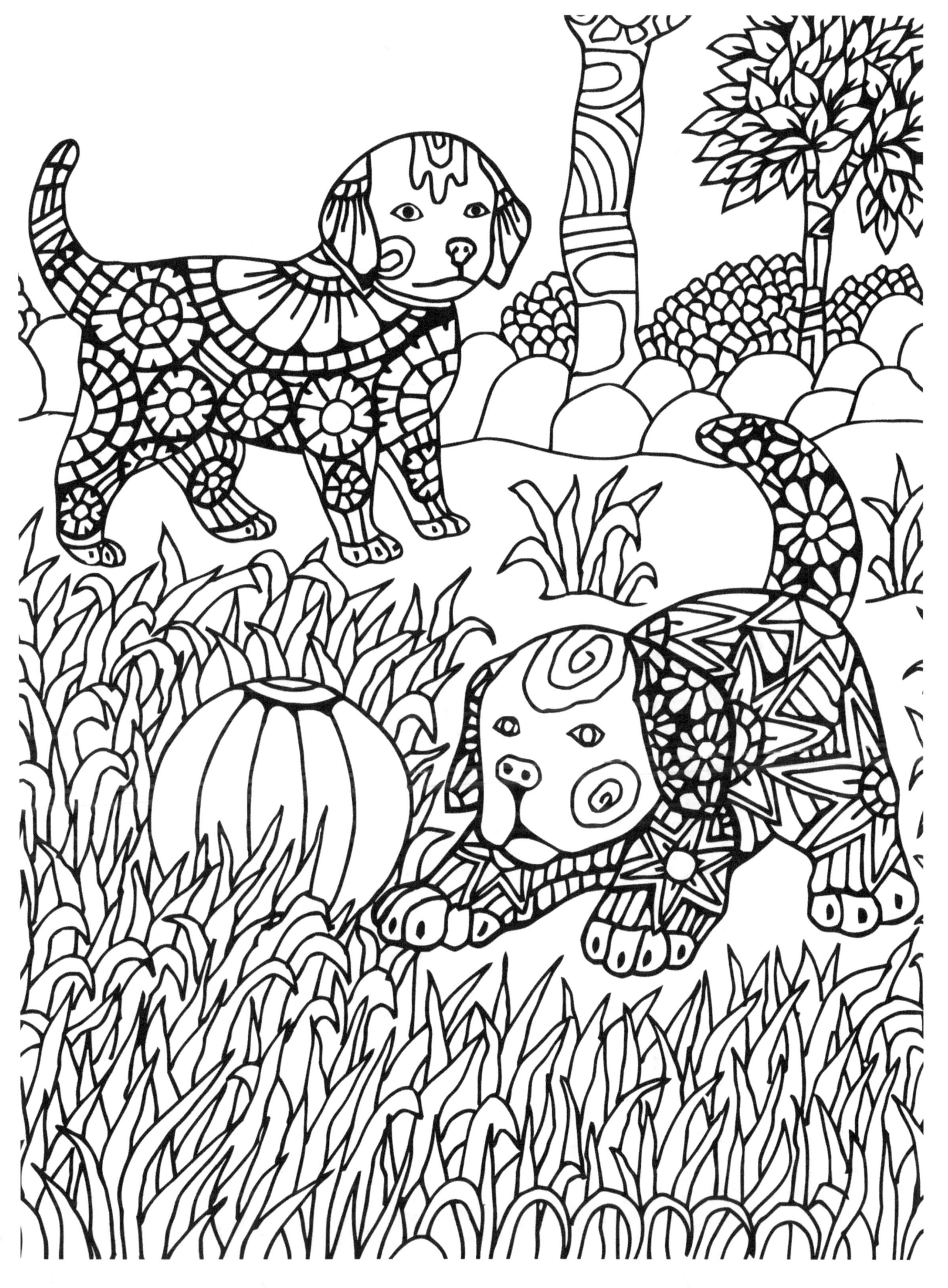

Left blank for your convenience

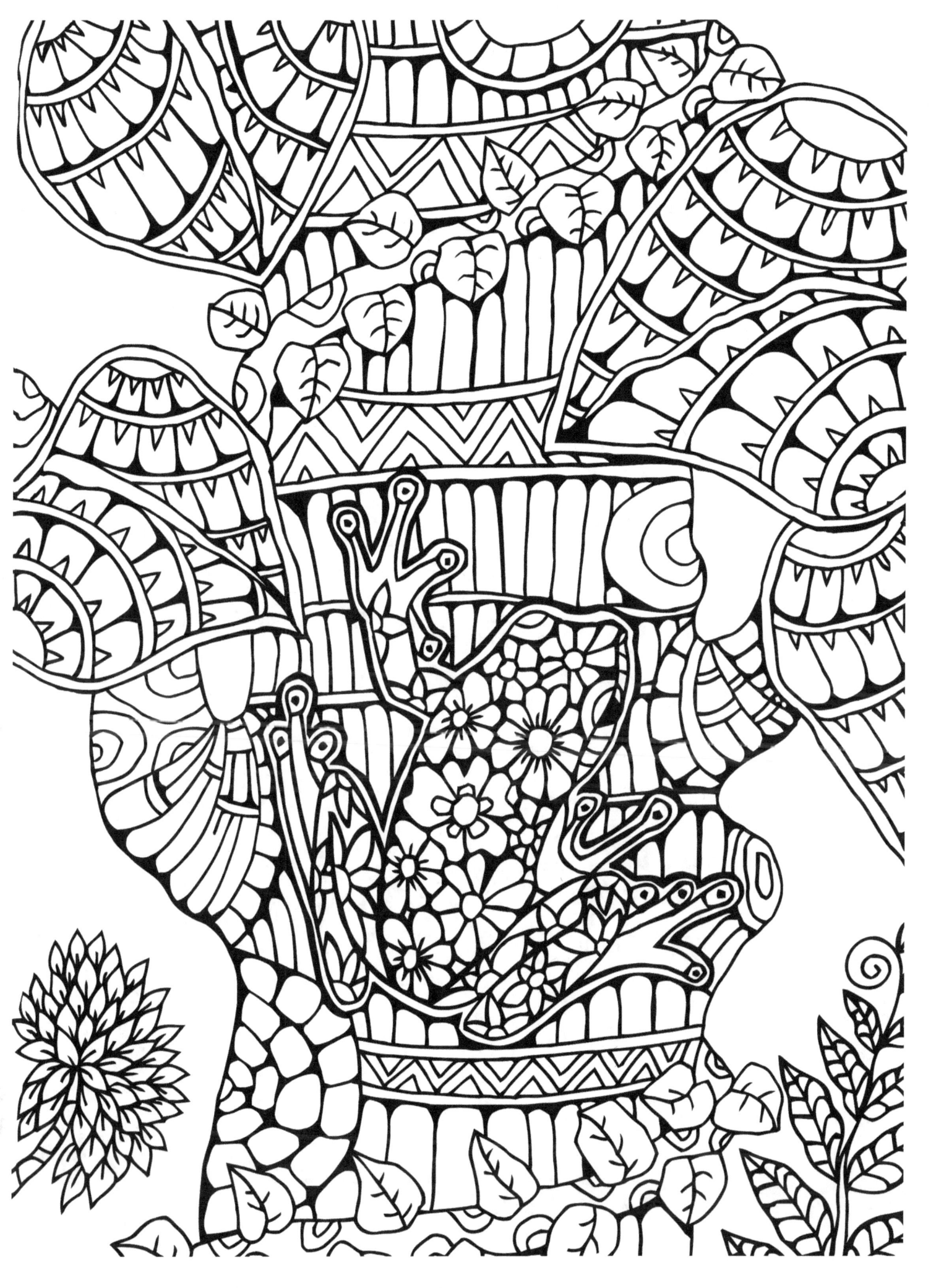

Left blank for your convenience

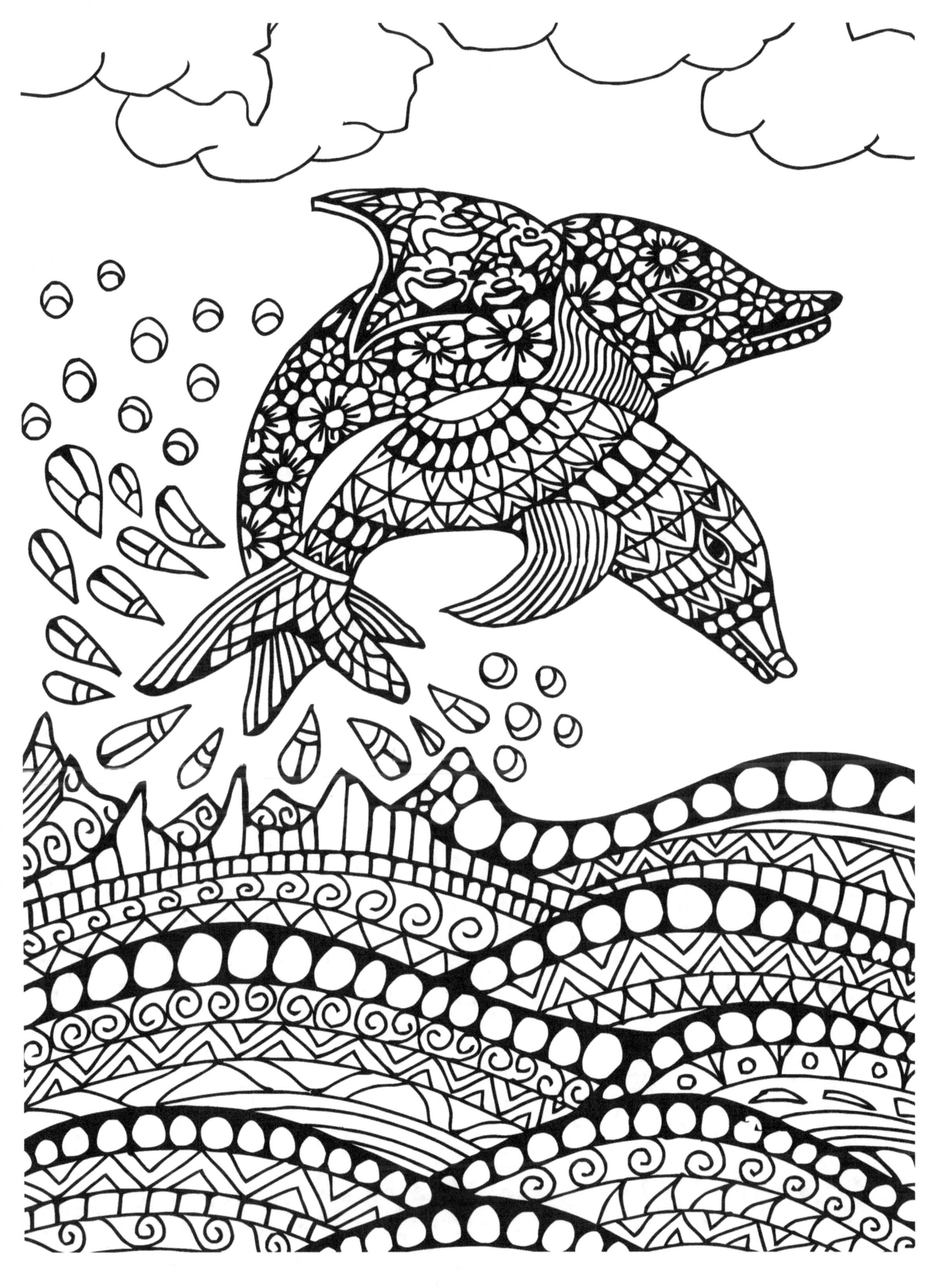

Left blank for your convenience

Left blank for your convenience

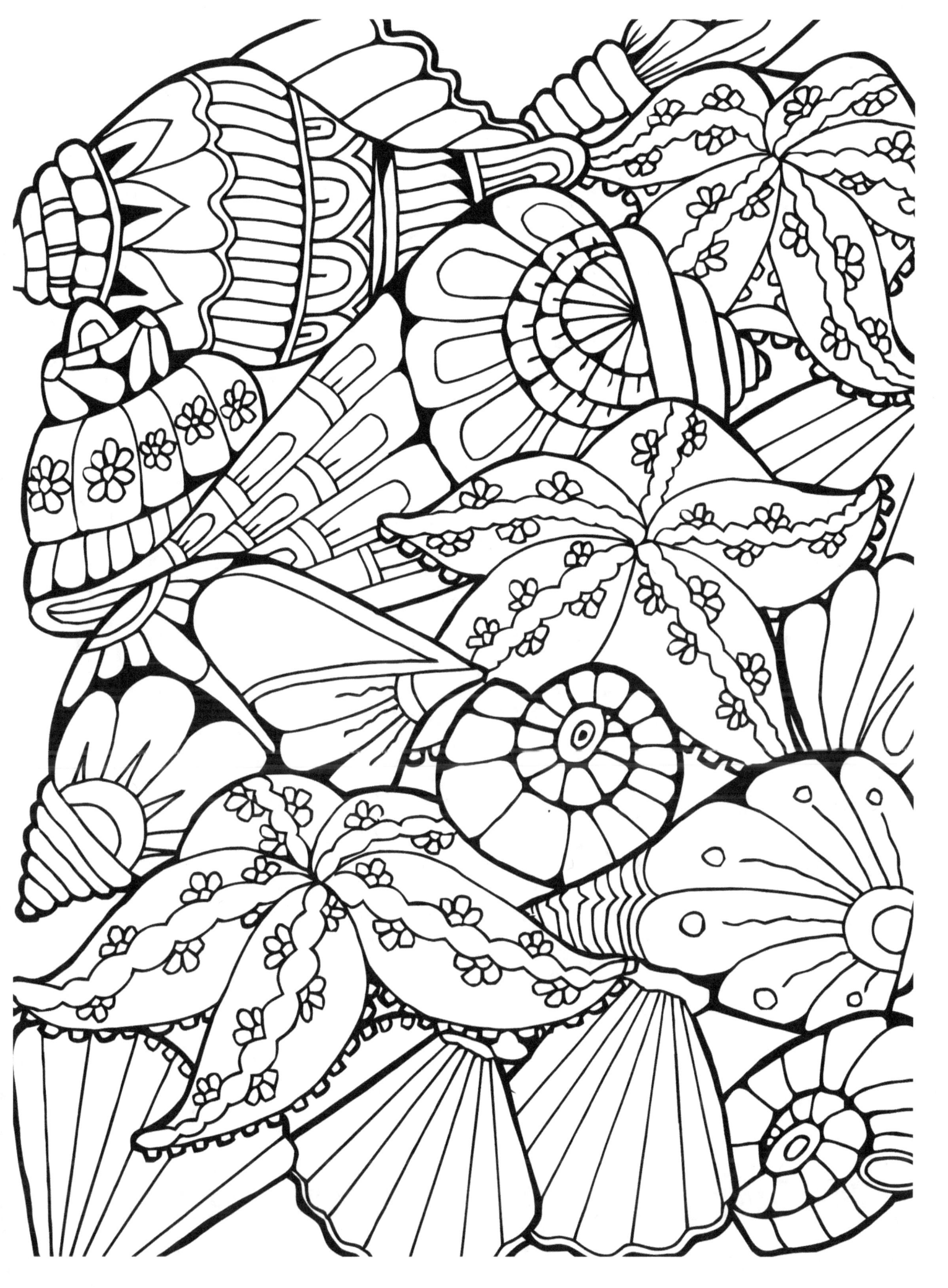

Left blank for your convenience

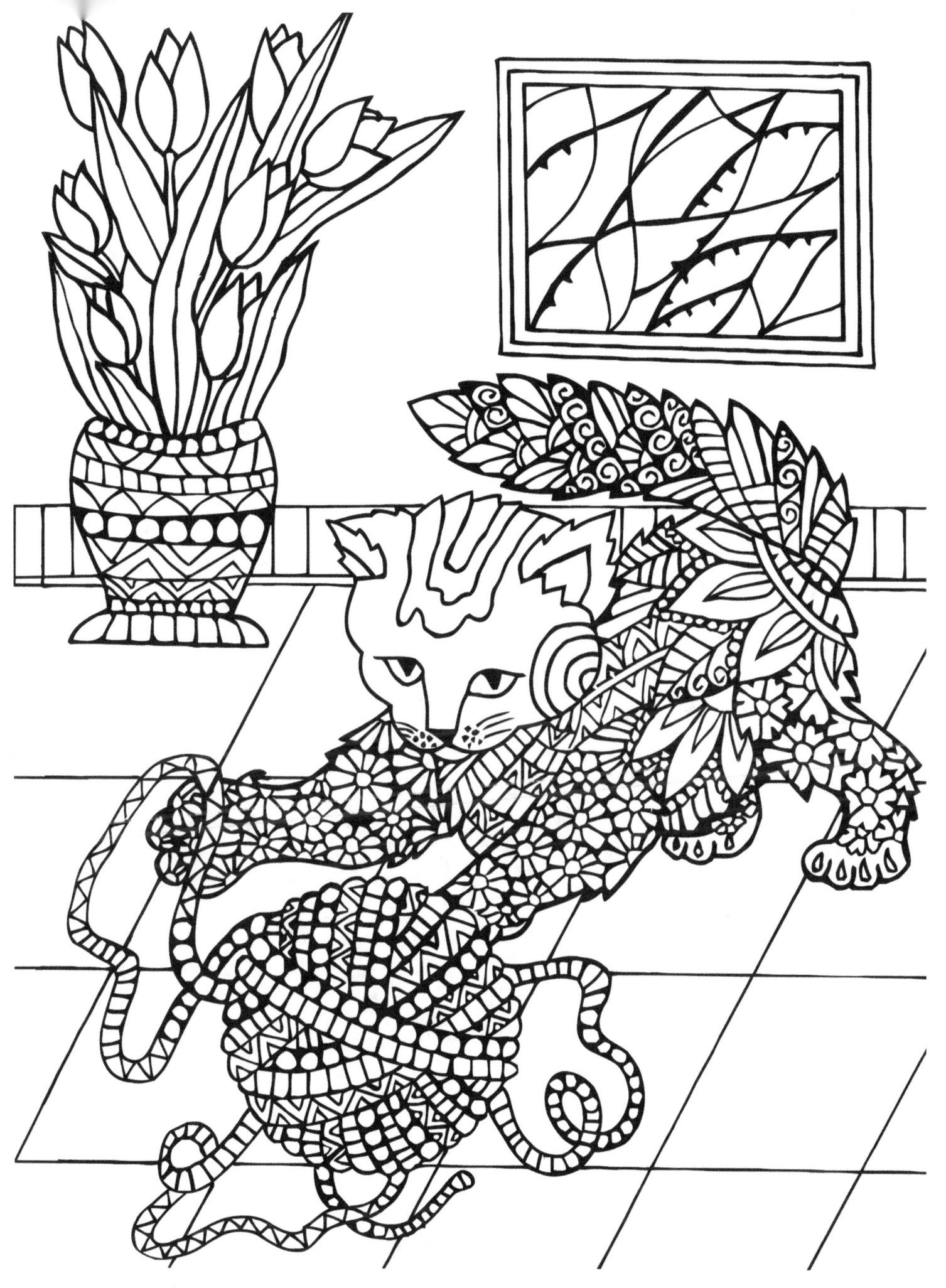

Left blank for your convenience

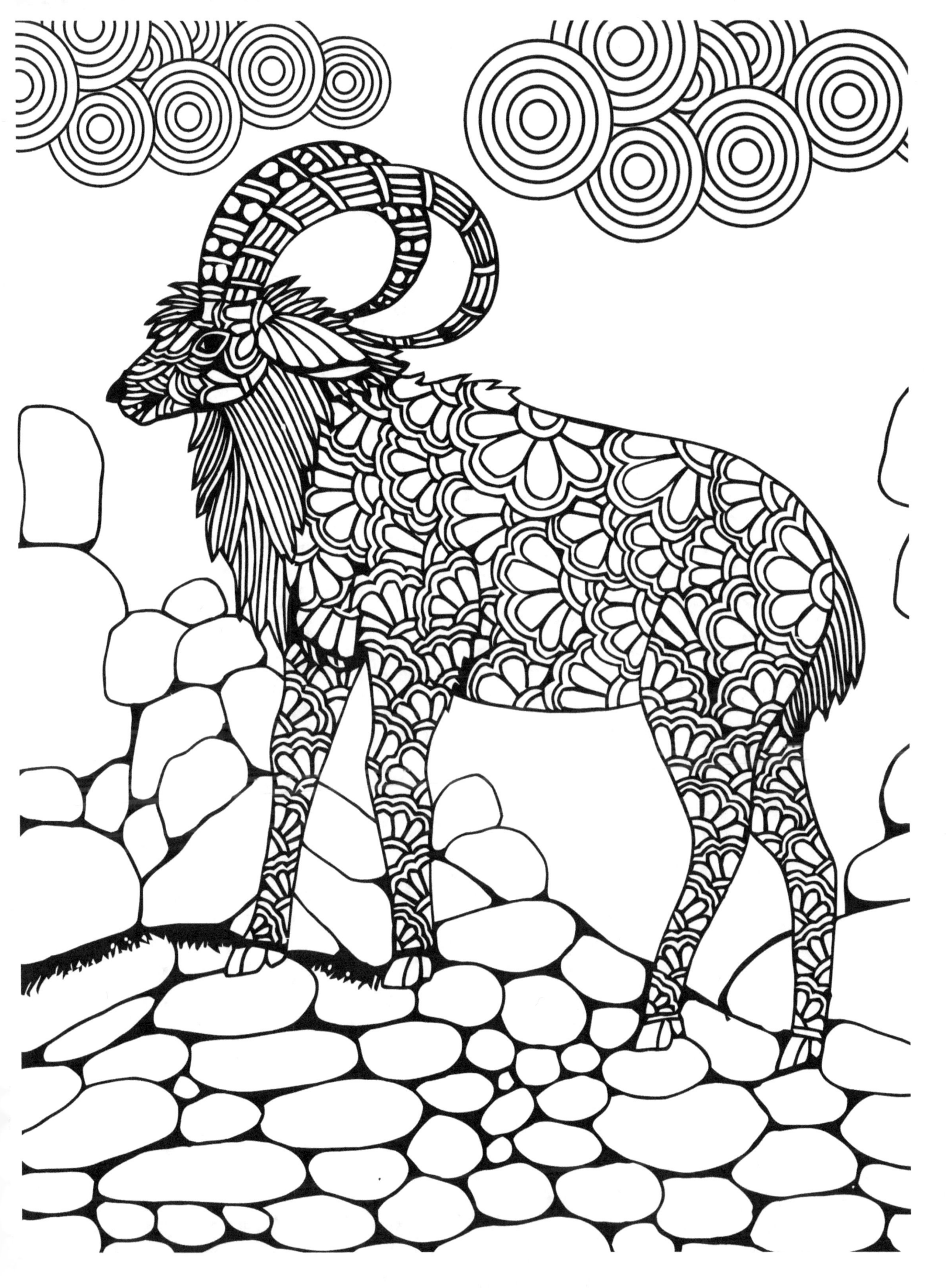

Left blank for your convenience

Left blank for your convenience

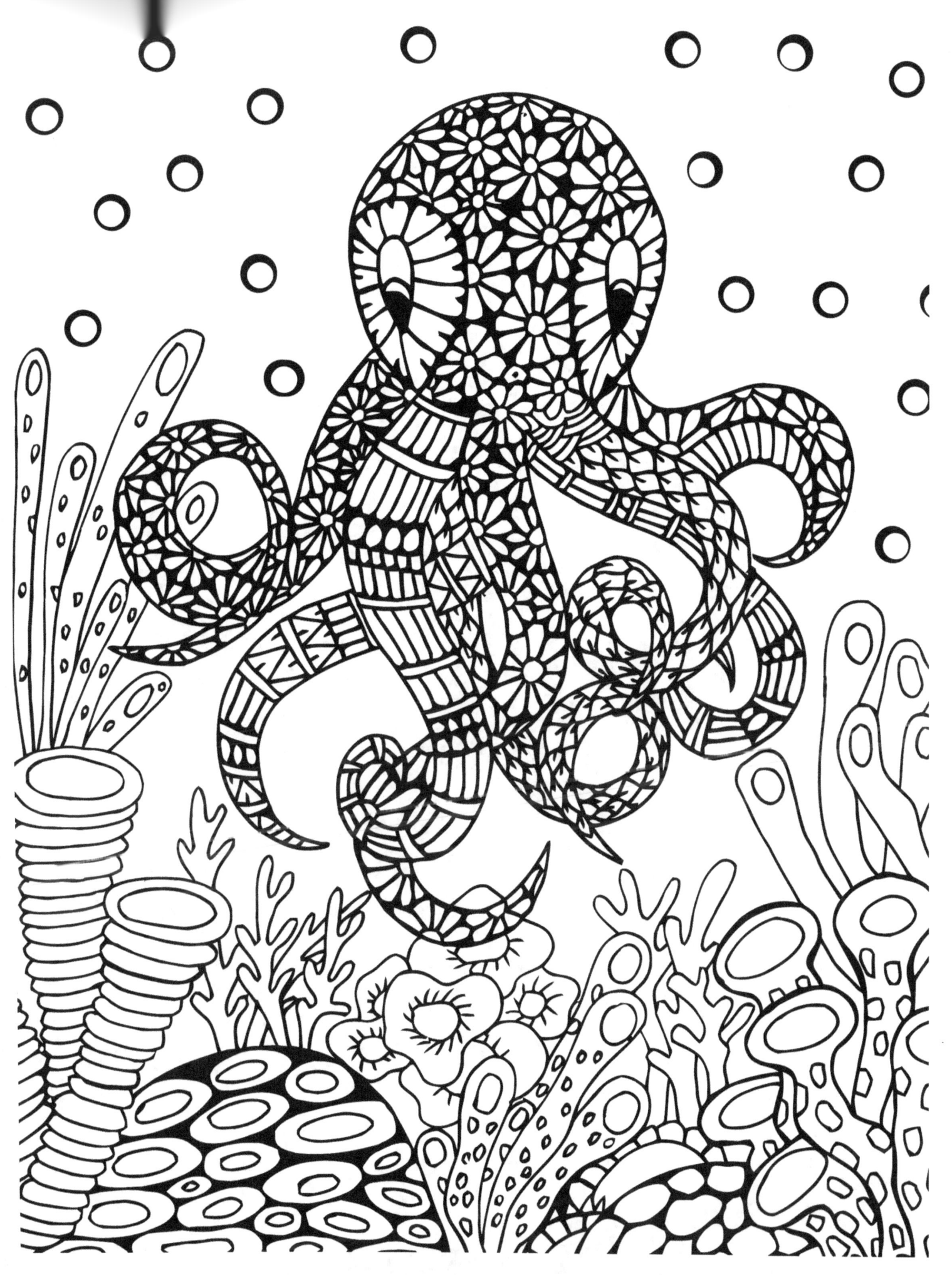

Left blank for your convenience

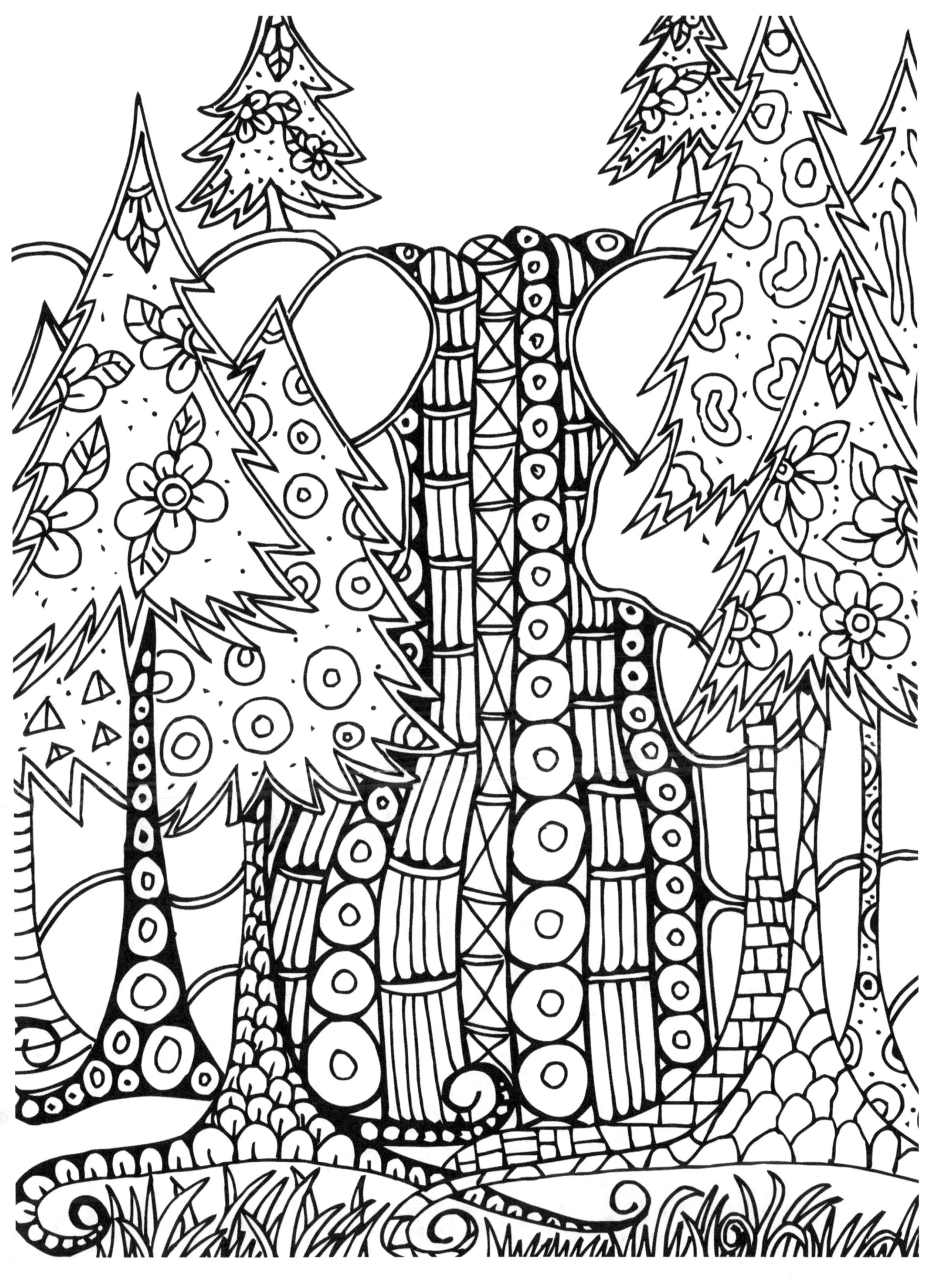

Left blank for your convenience

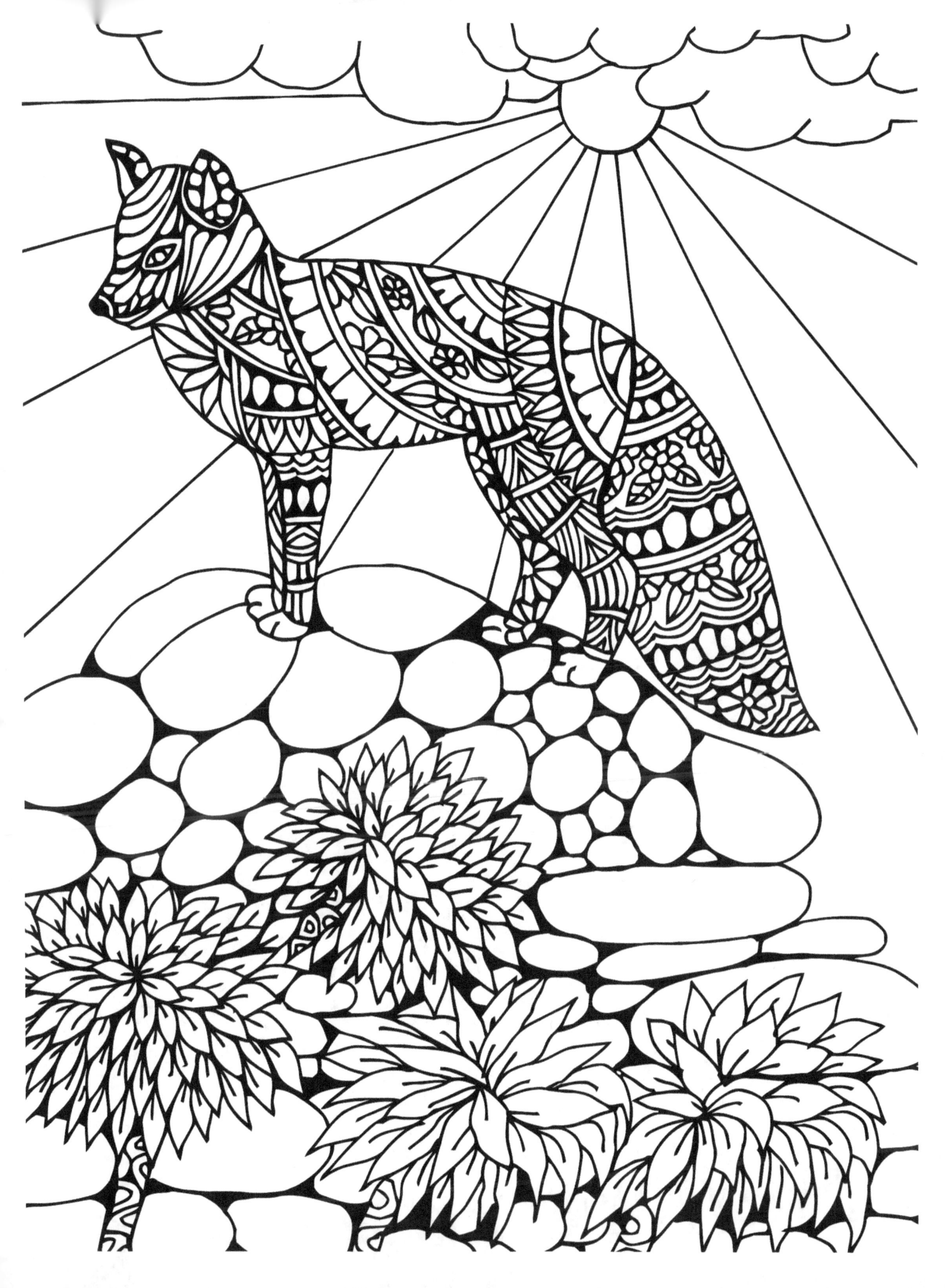

Left blank for your convenience

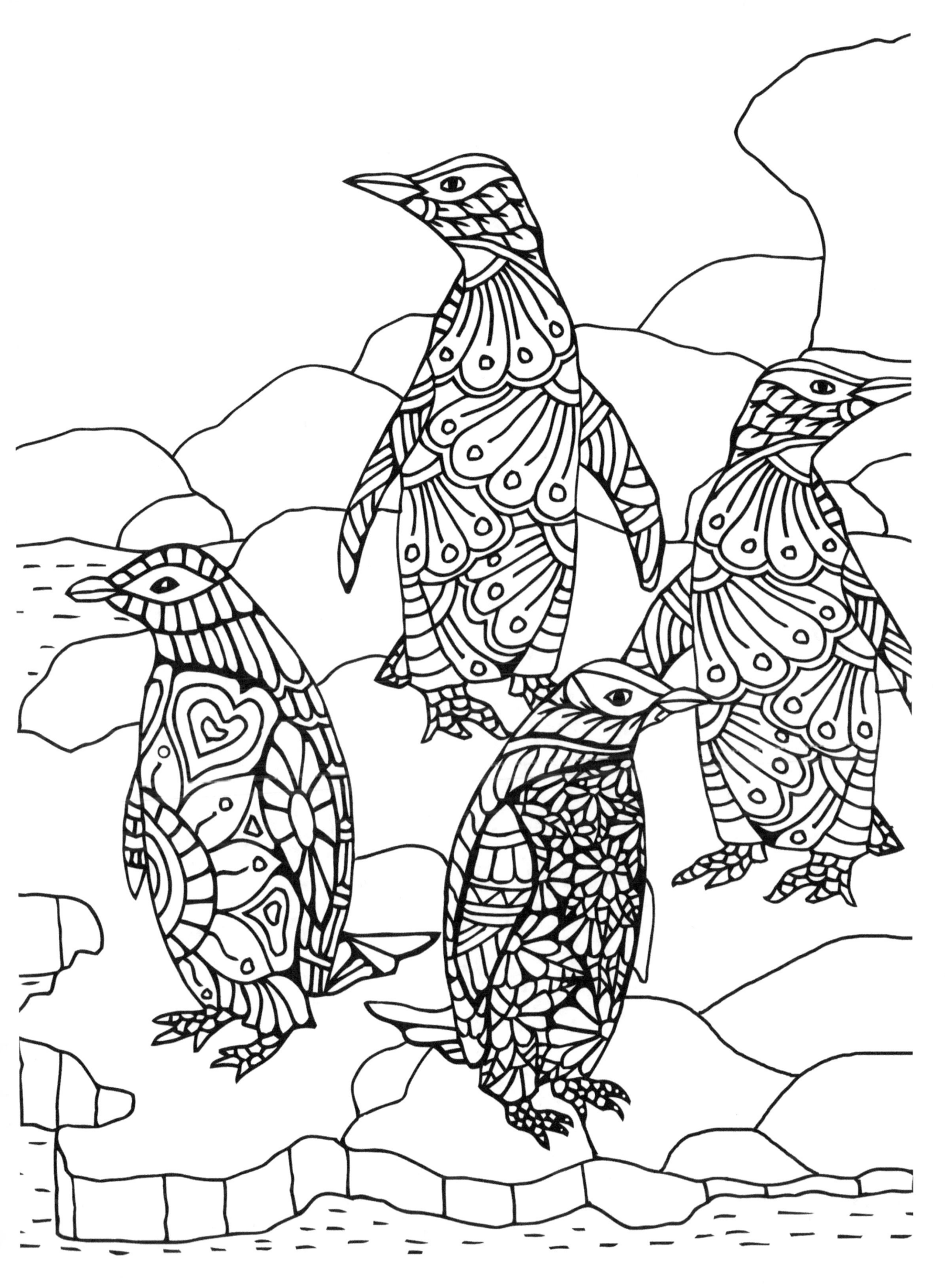

Left blank for your convenience

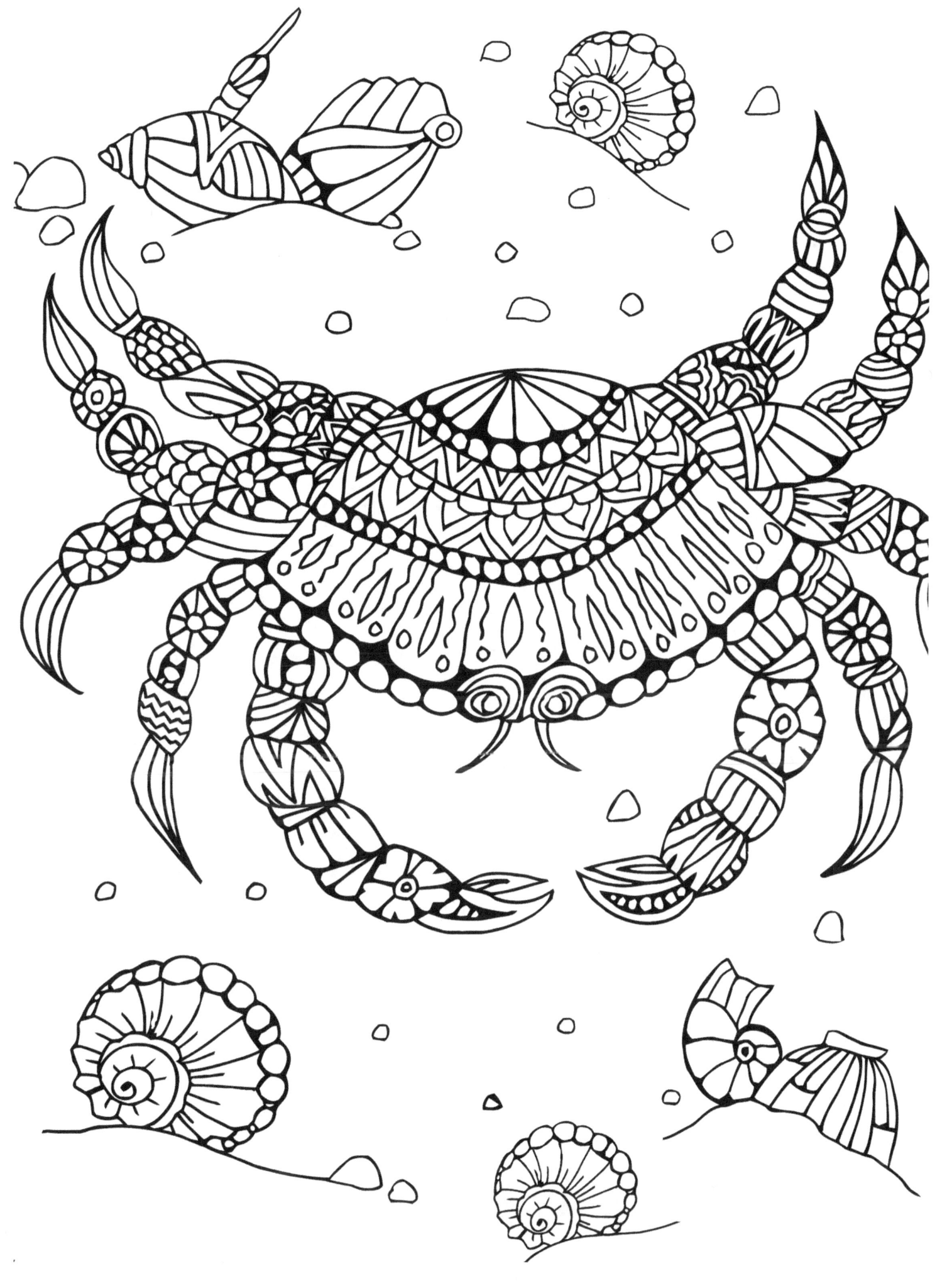

Left blank for your convenience

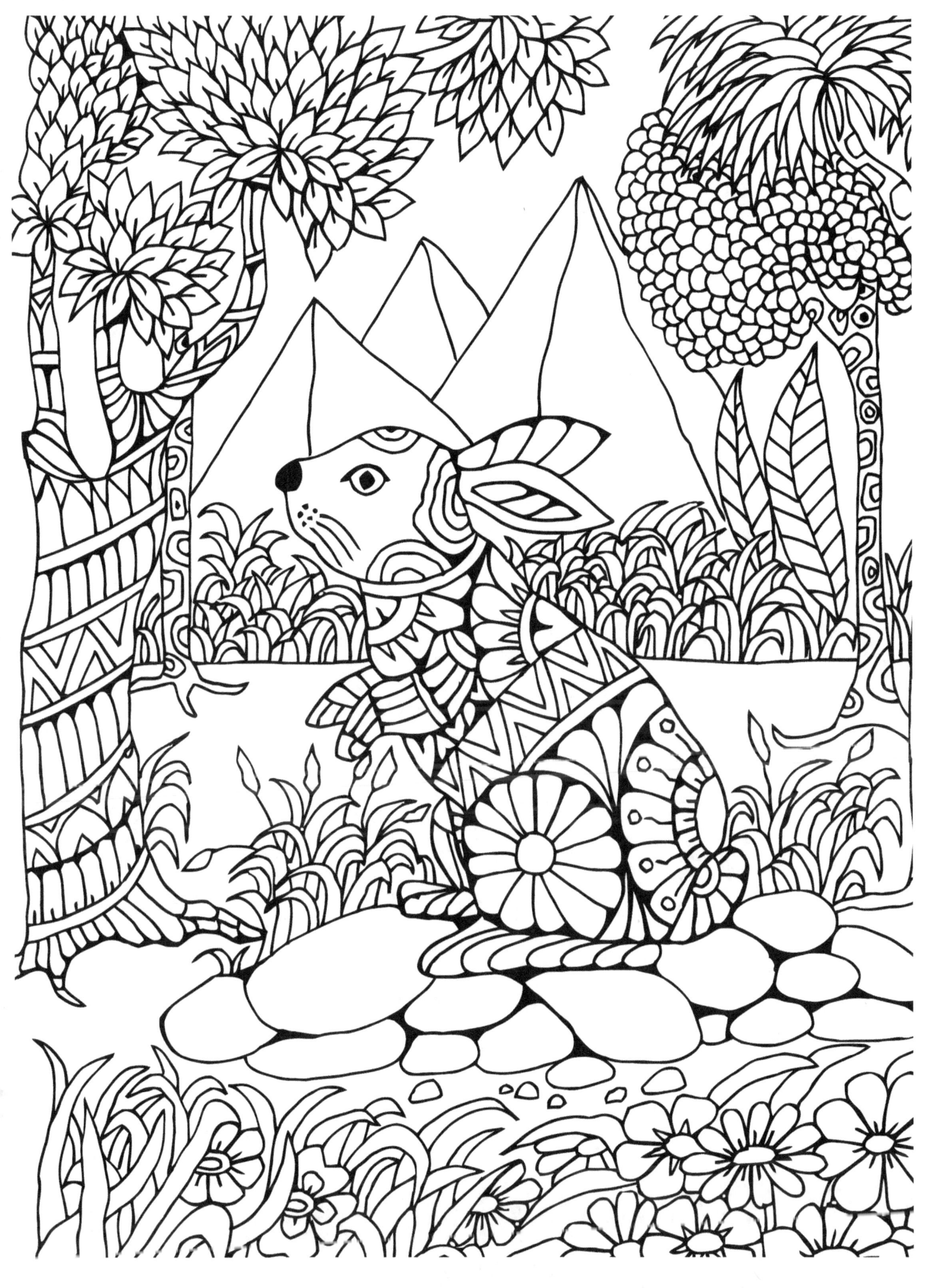

Left blank for your convenience

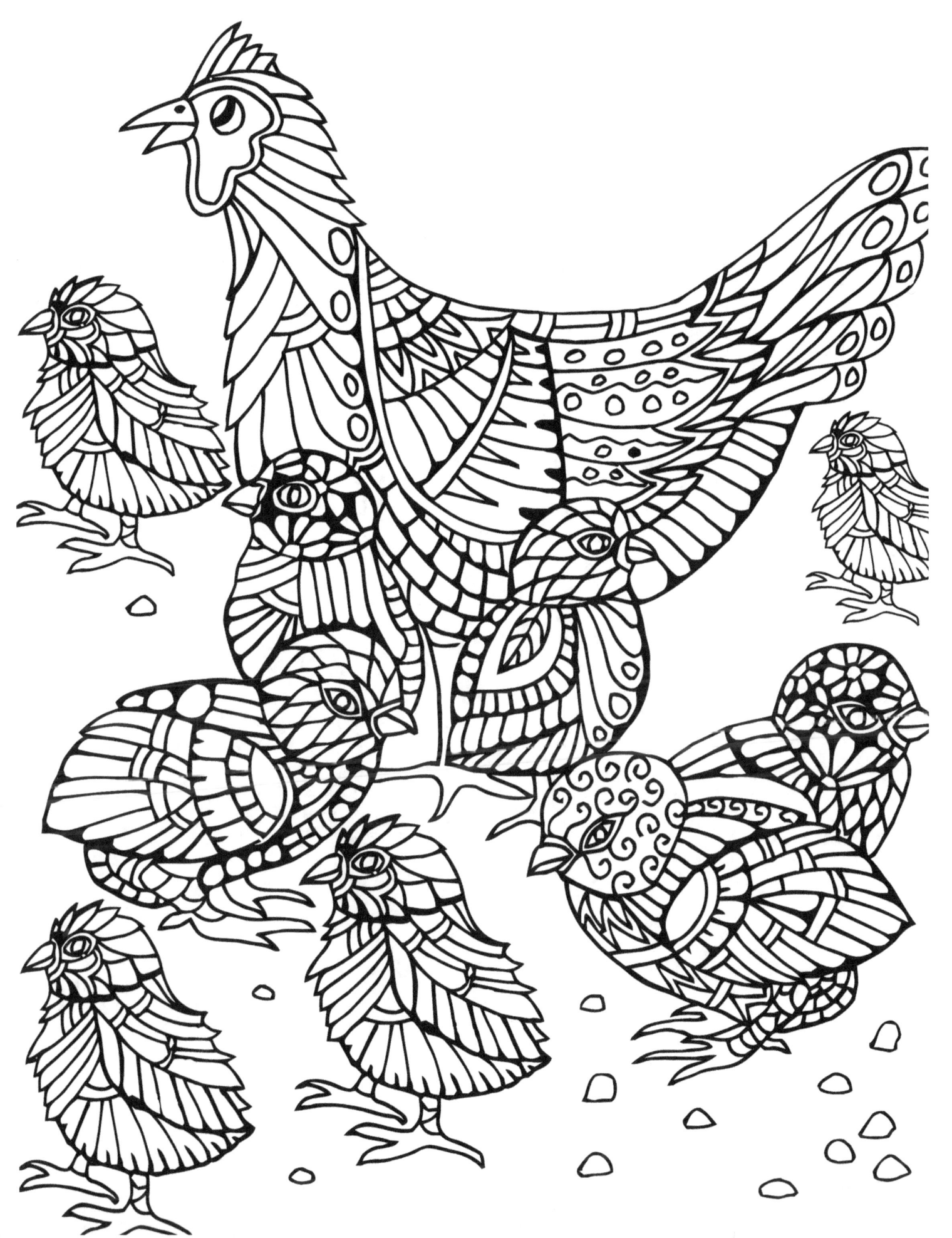

Left blank for your convenience

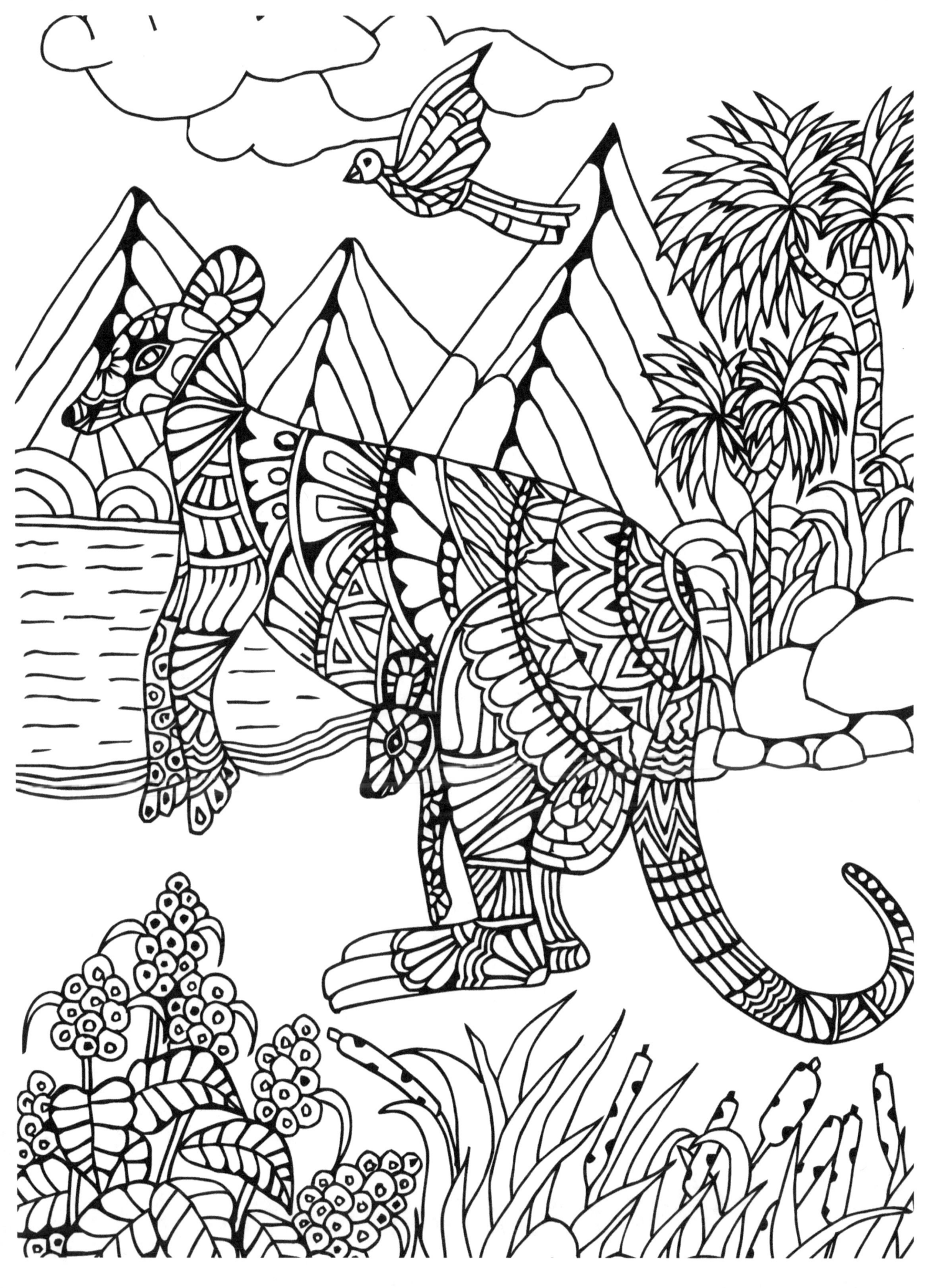

Left blank for your convenience

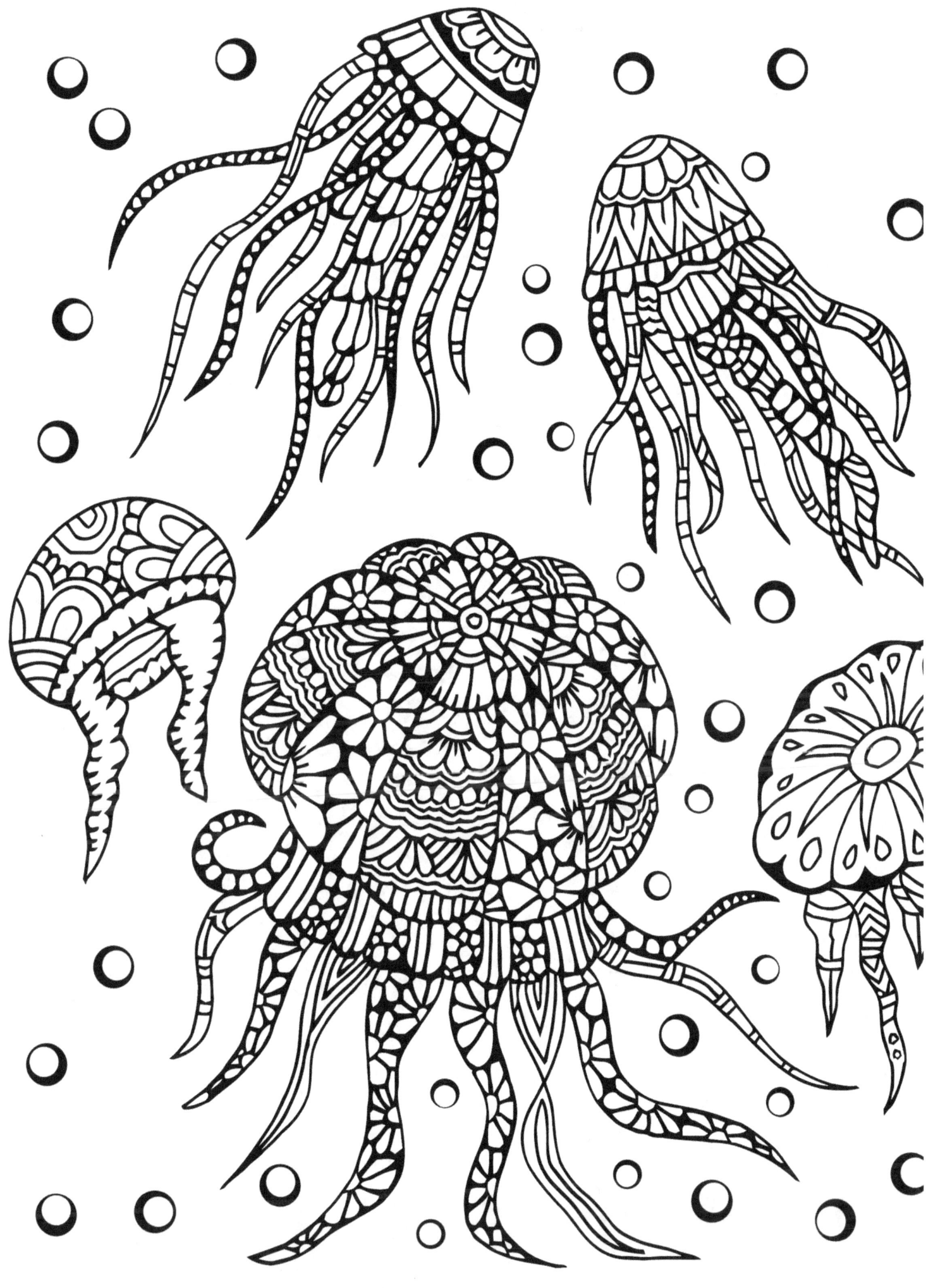

Left blank for your convenience

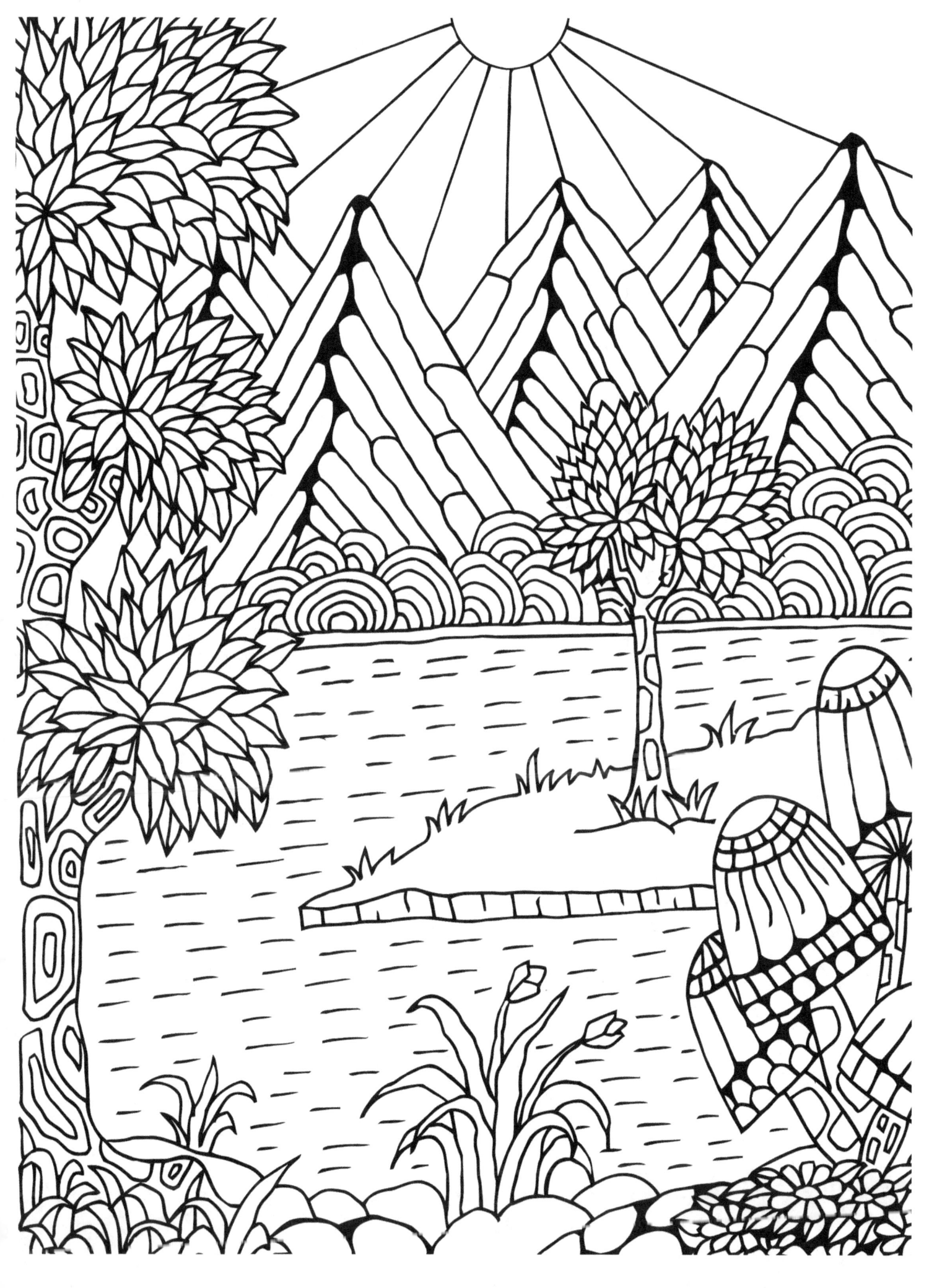

Left blank for your convenience

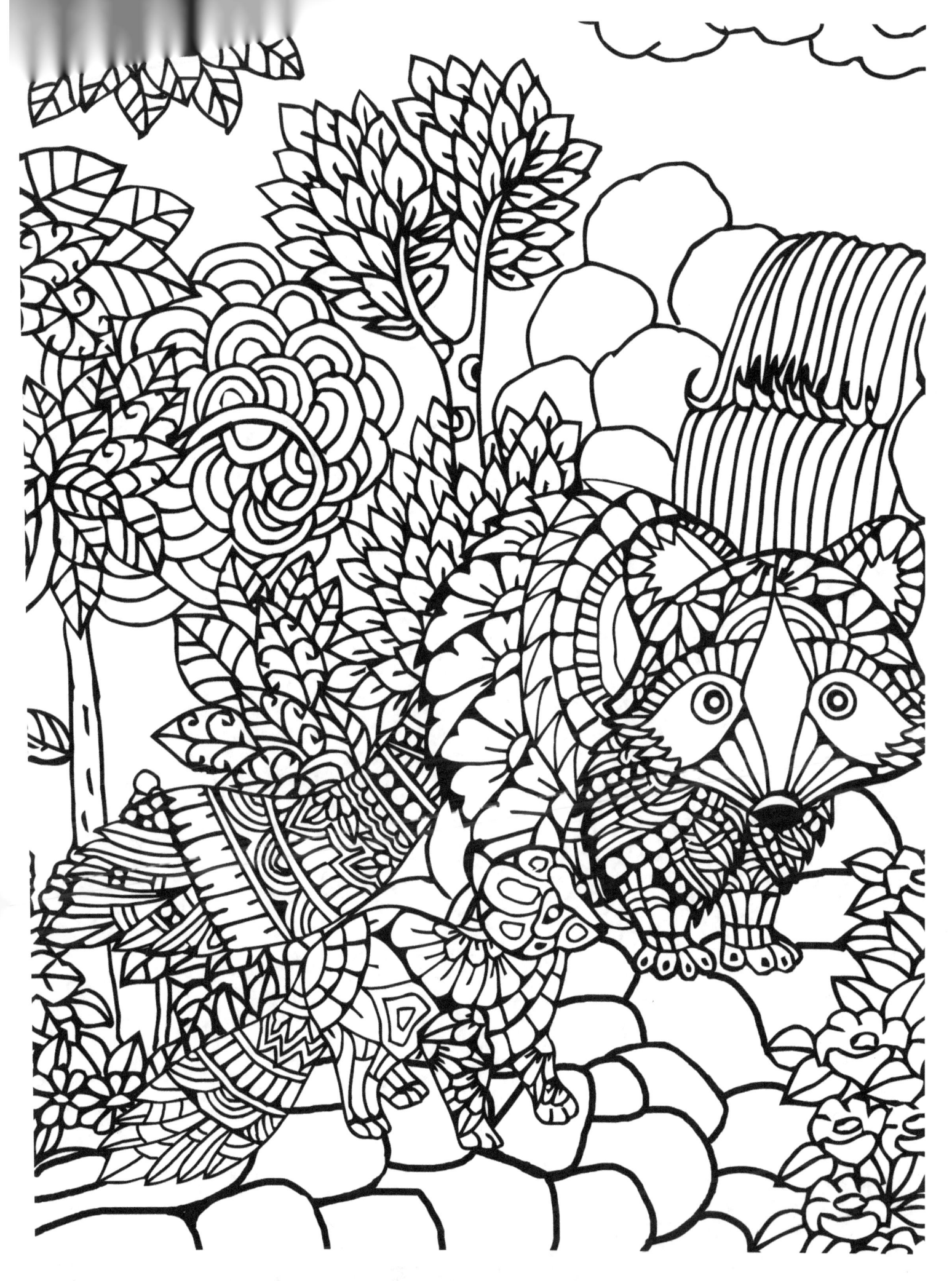

Left blank for your convenience

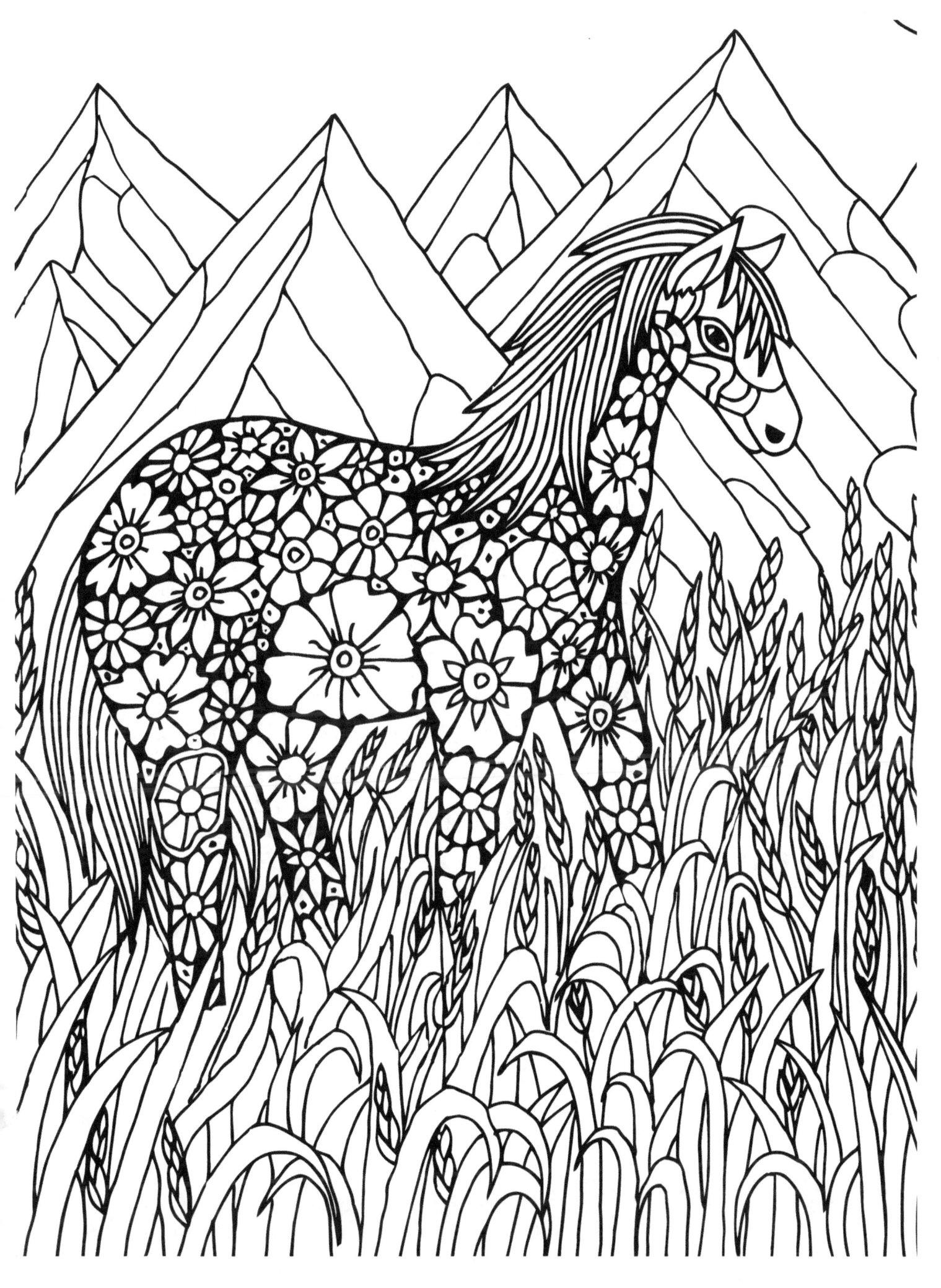

Left blank for your convenience

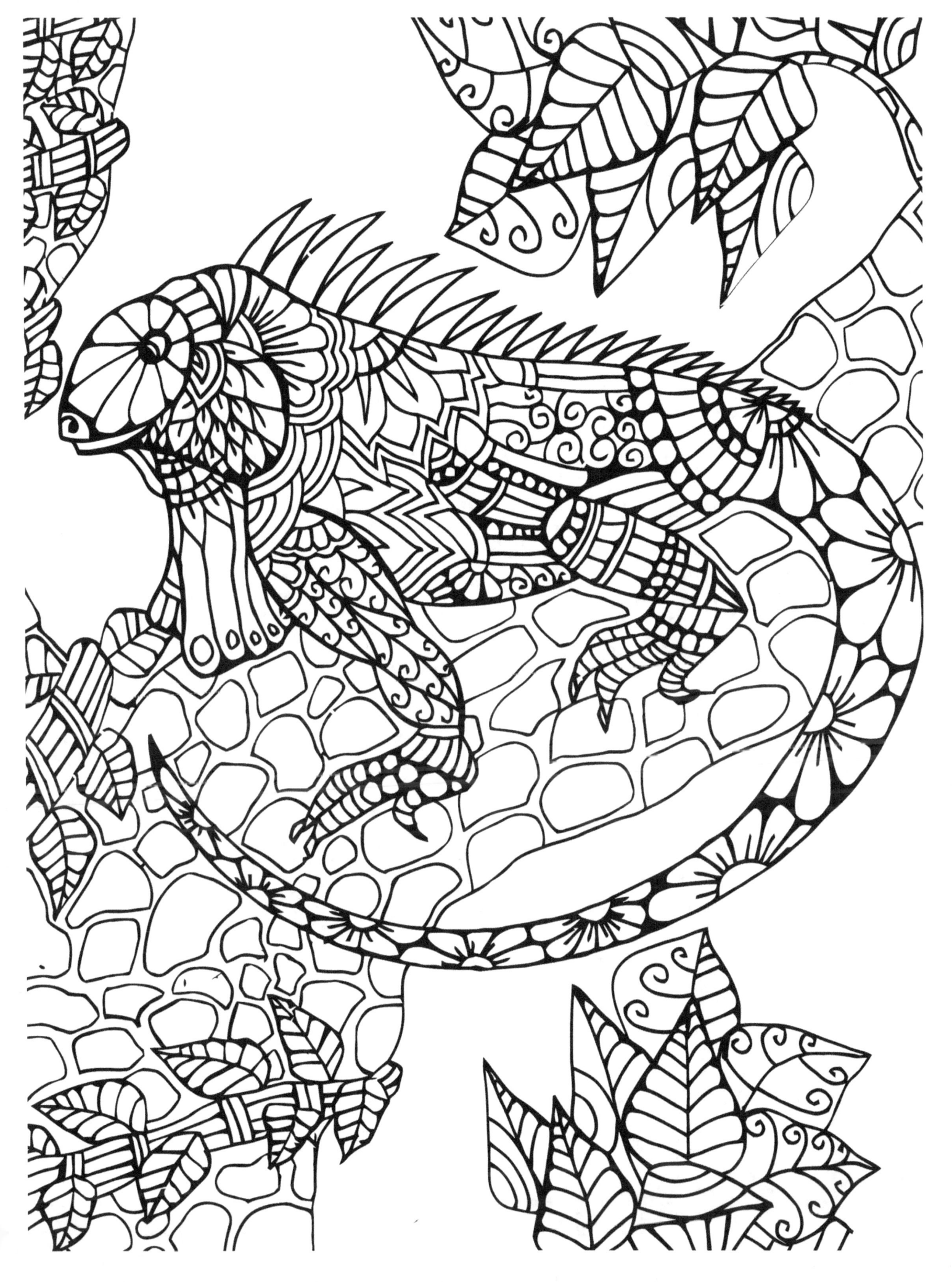

Left blank for your convenience

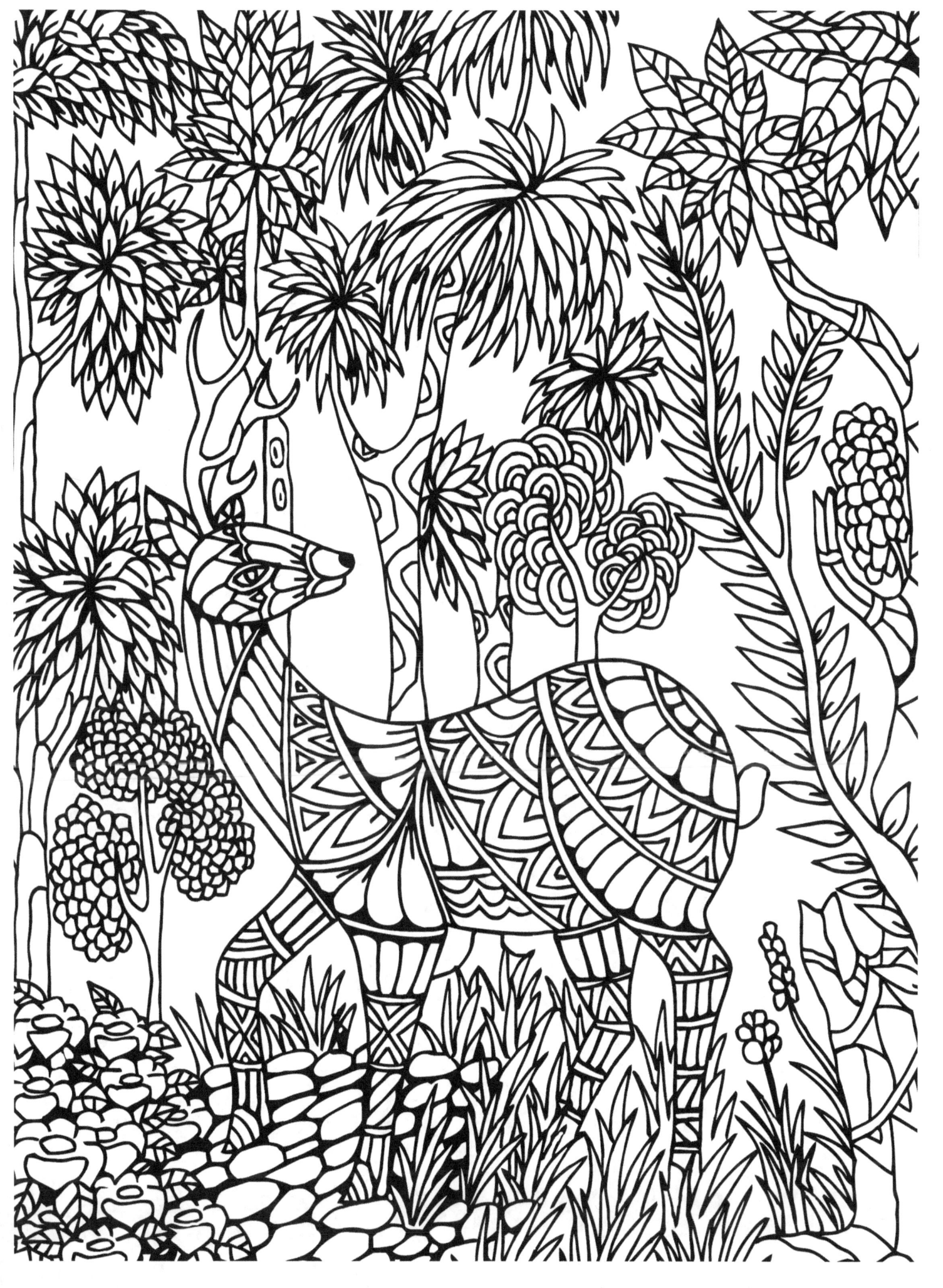

Left blank for your convenience

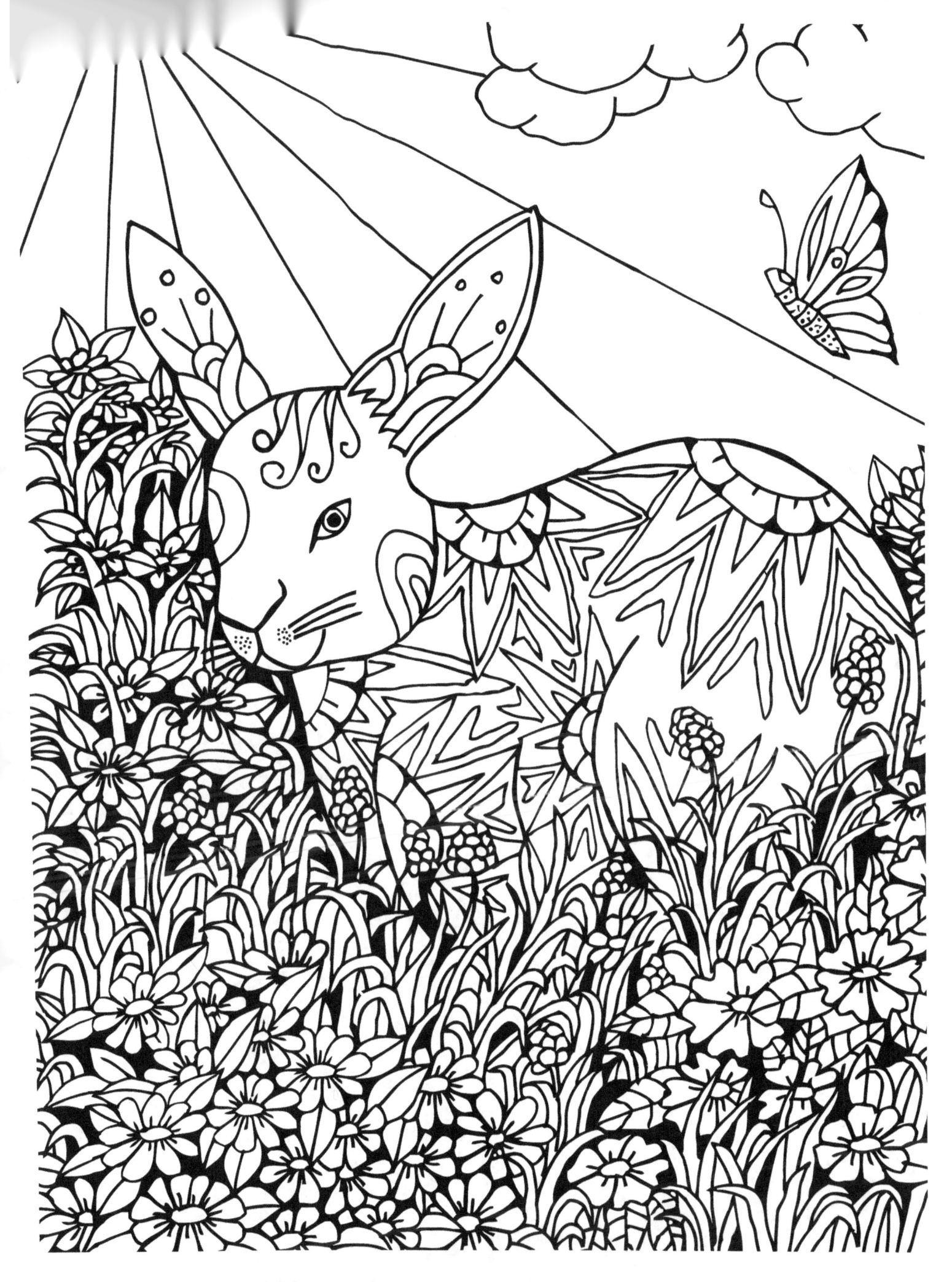

Left blank for your convenience

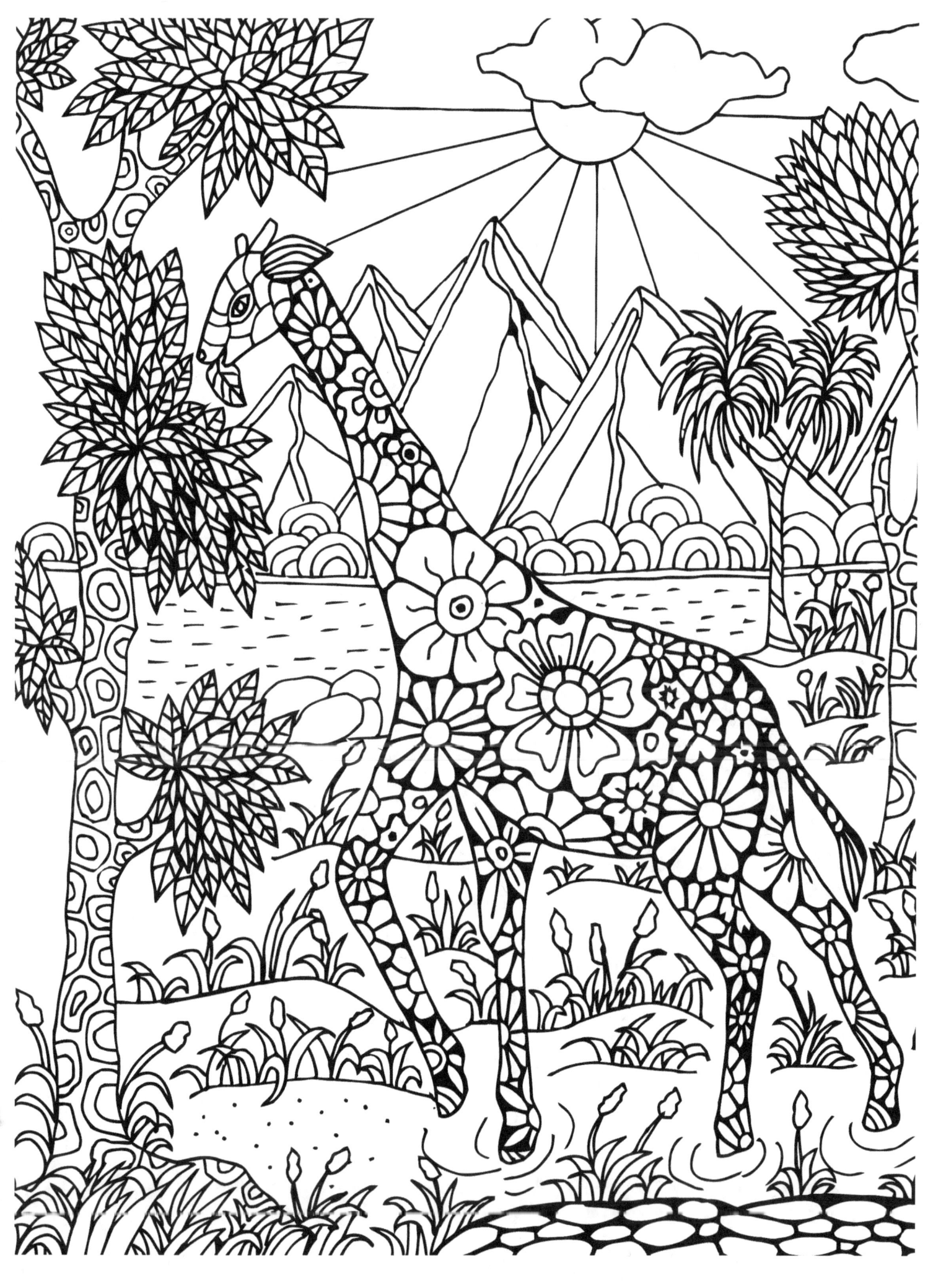

Left blank for your convenience

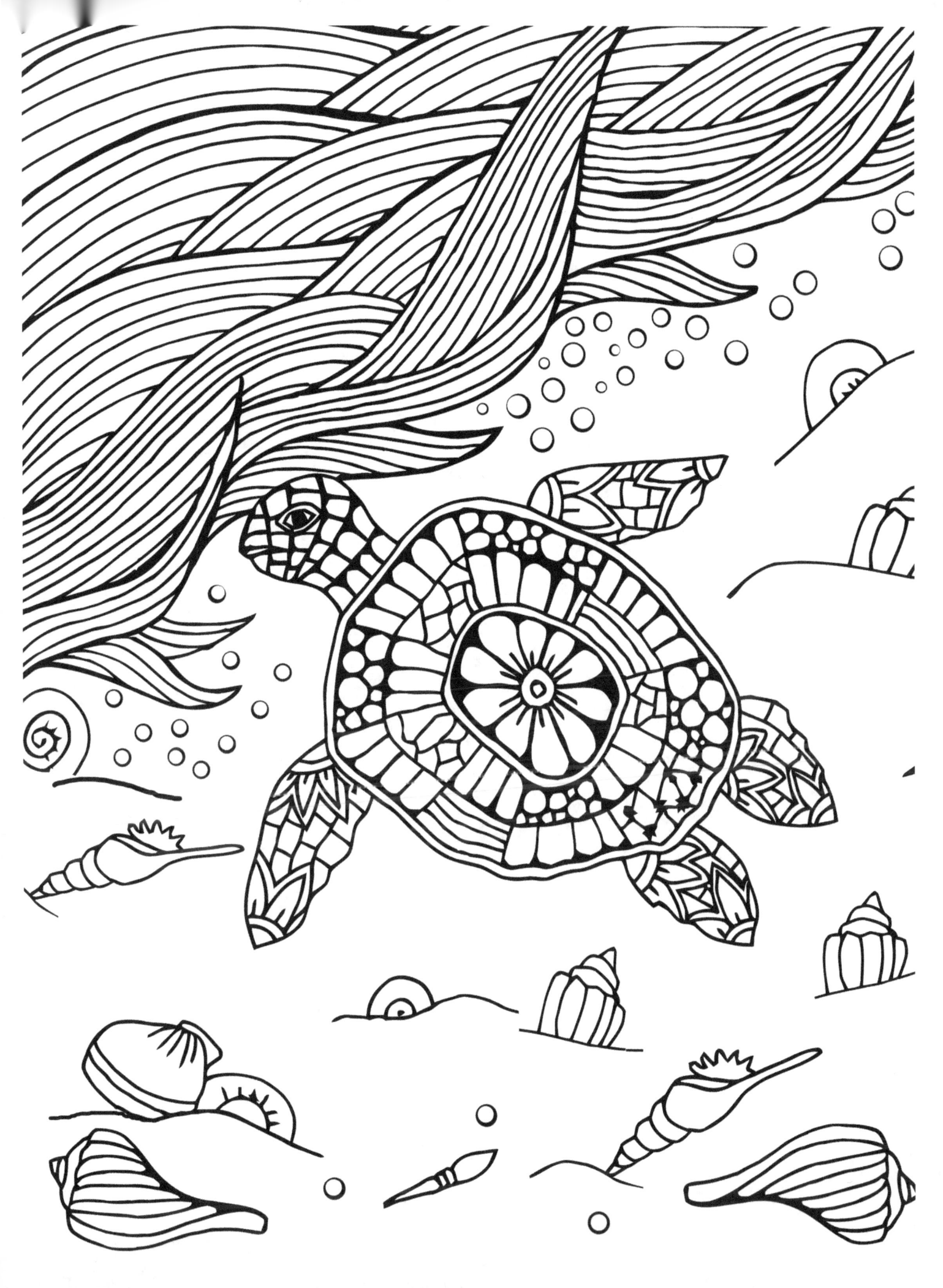

Left blank for your convenience

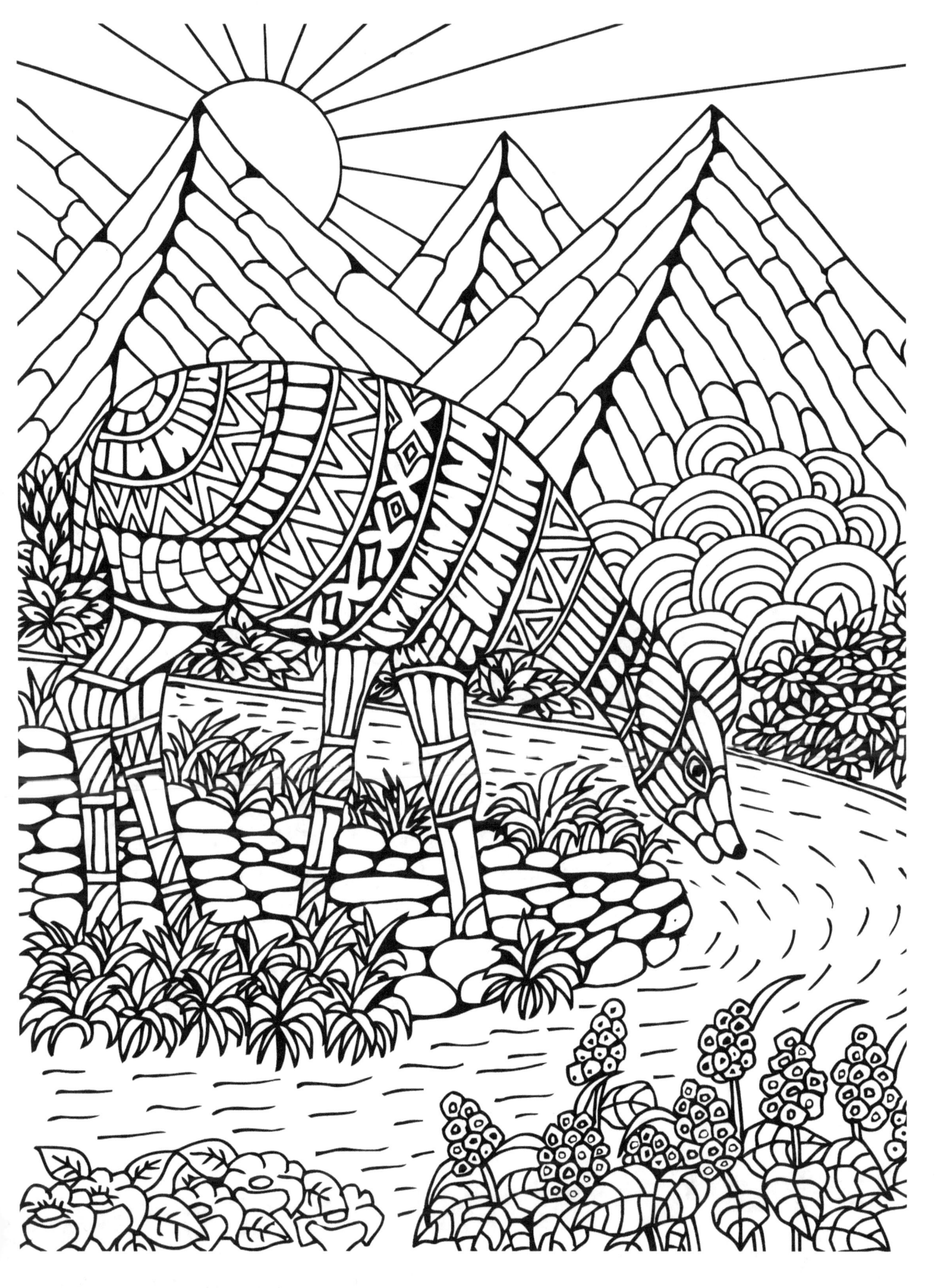

Left blank for your convenience

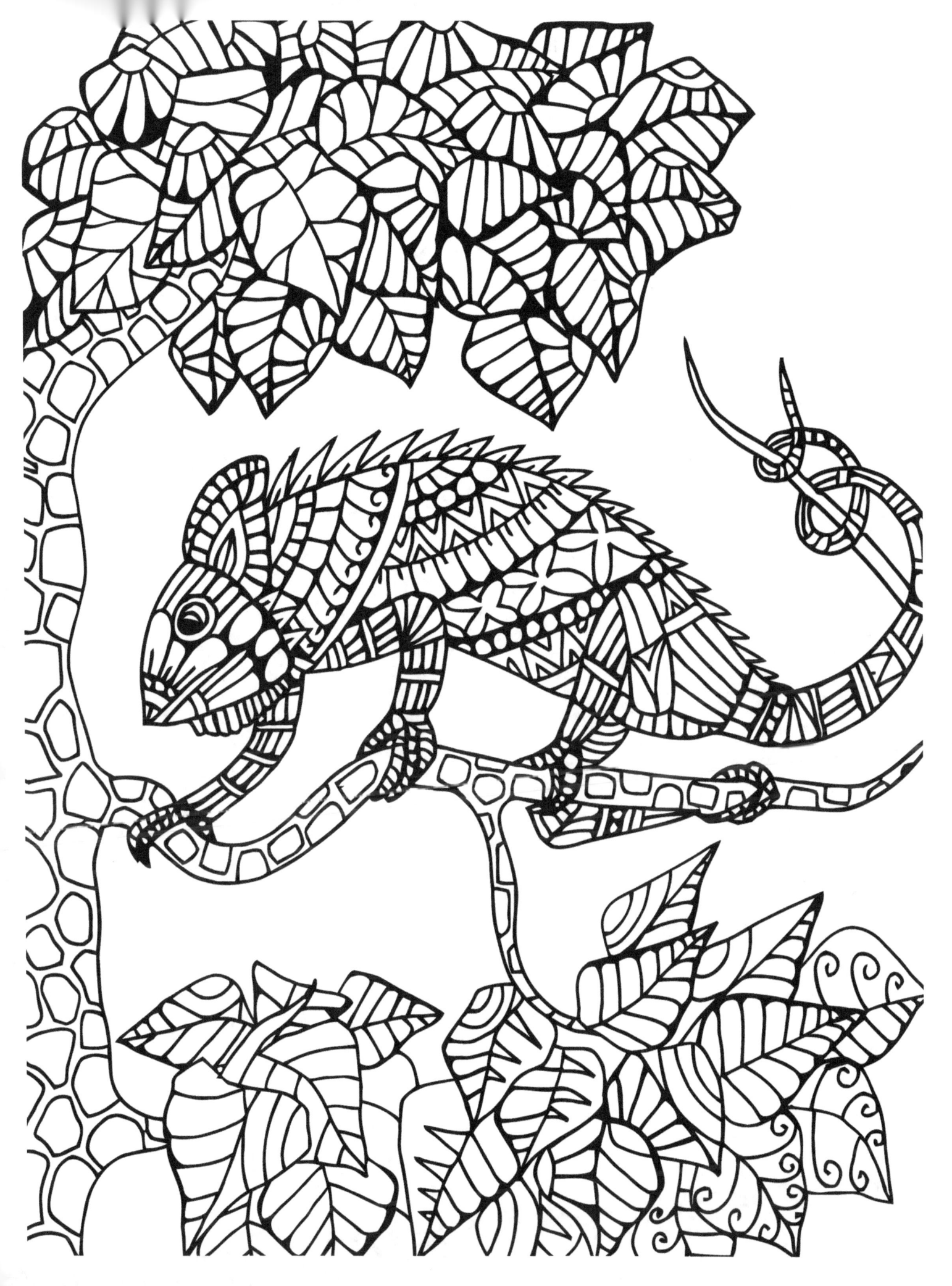

Left blank for your convenience

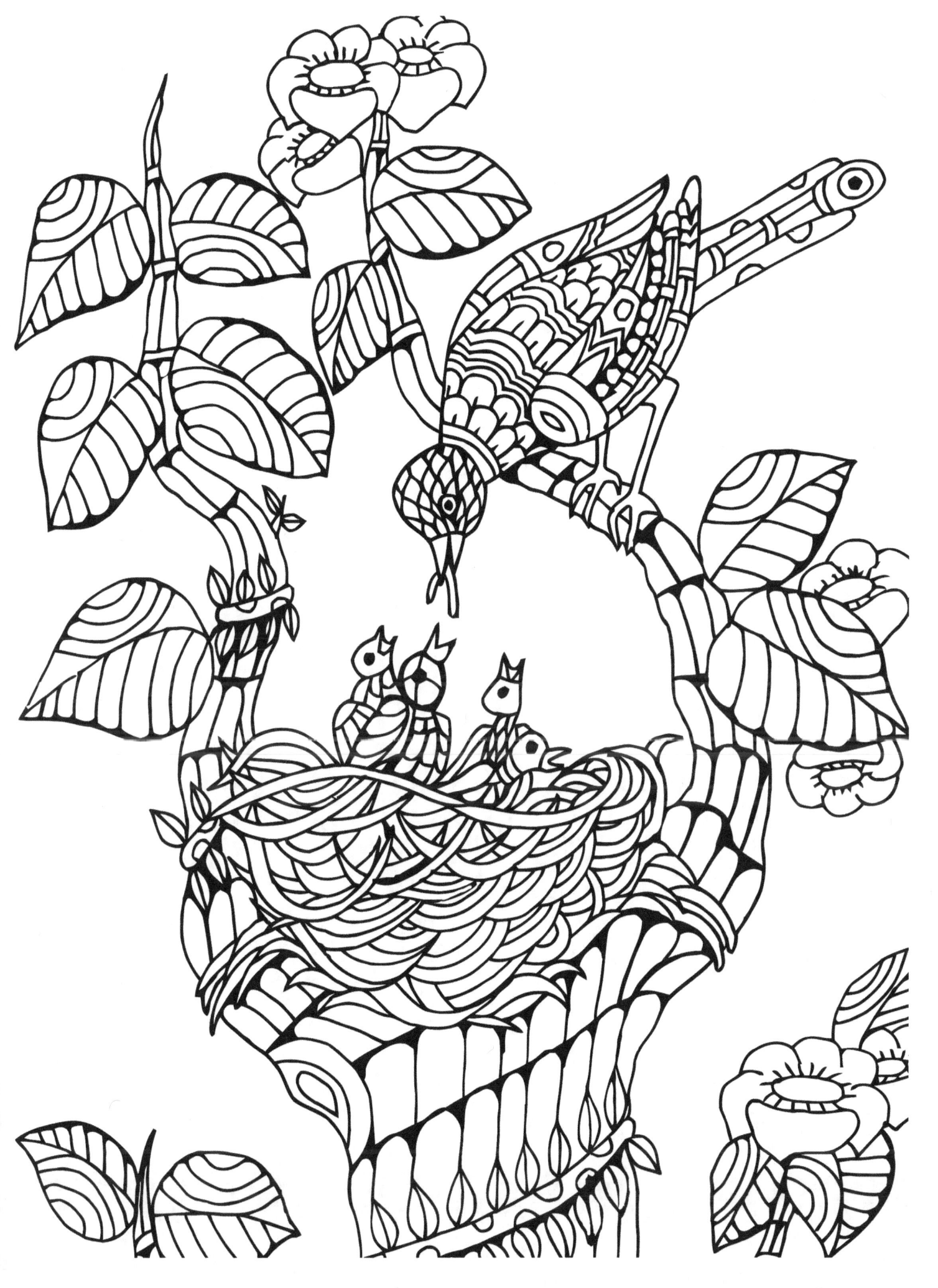

Left blank for your convenience

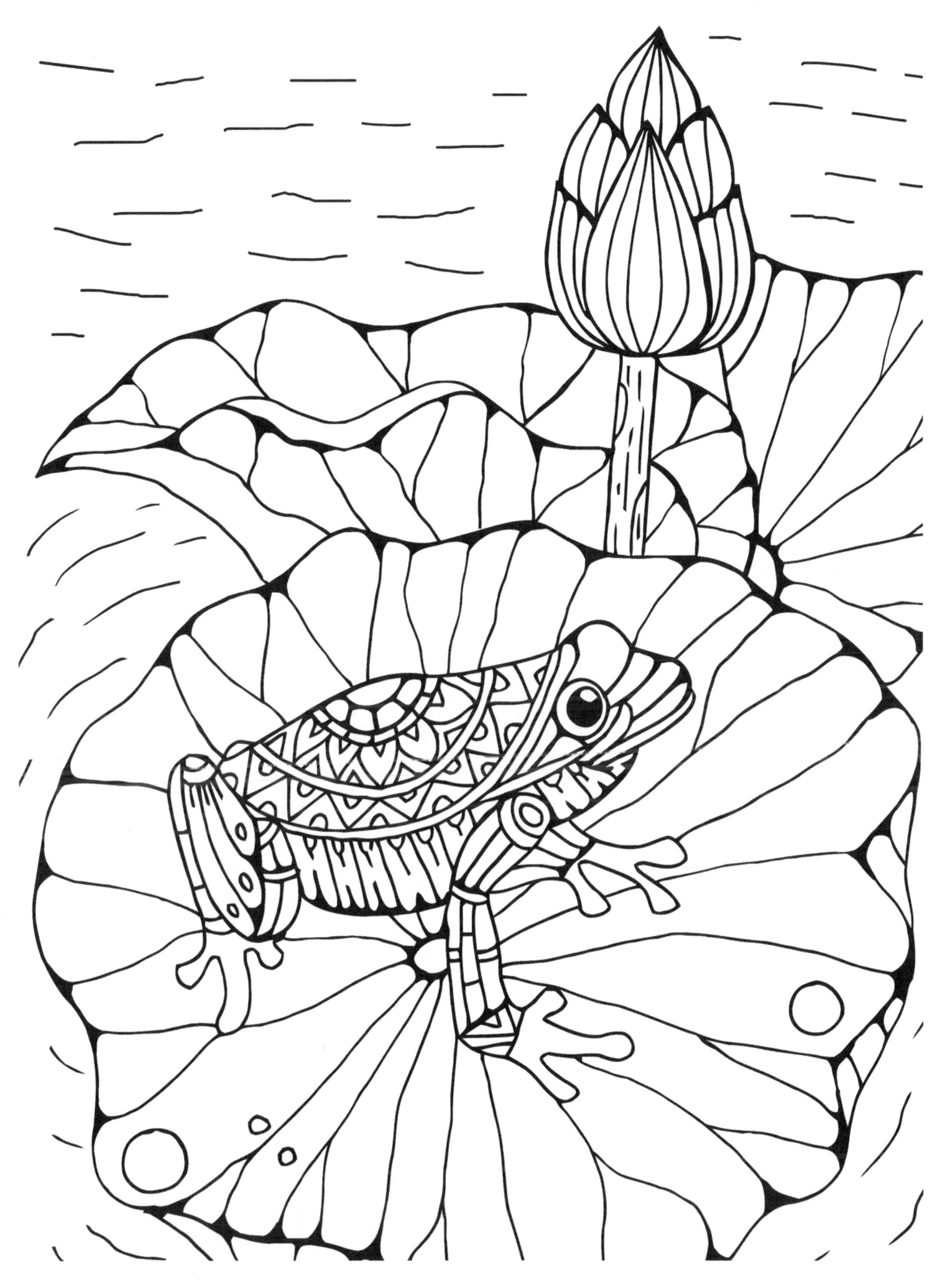

Left blank for your convenience

Left blank for your convenience

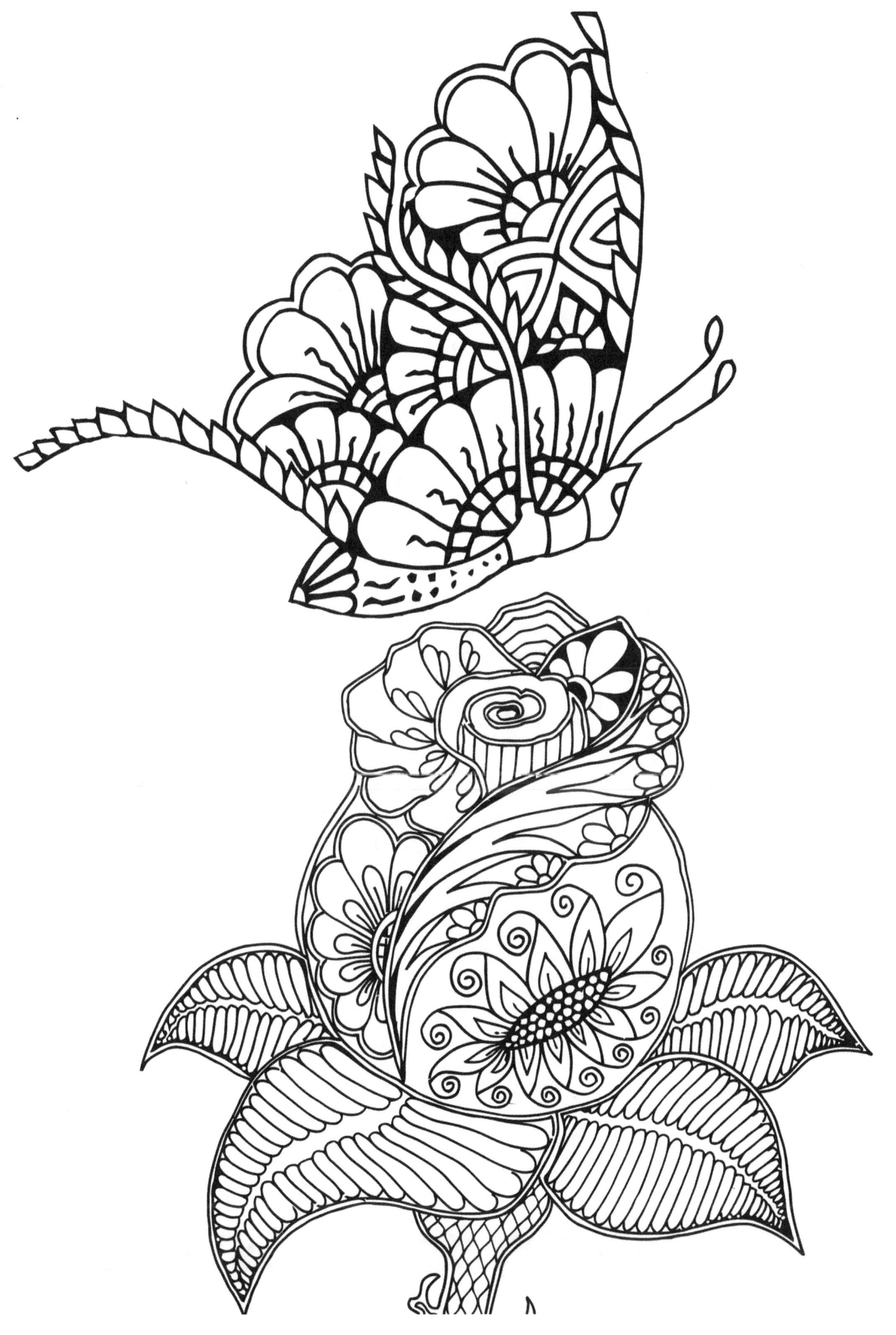

Left blank for your convenience

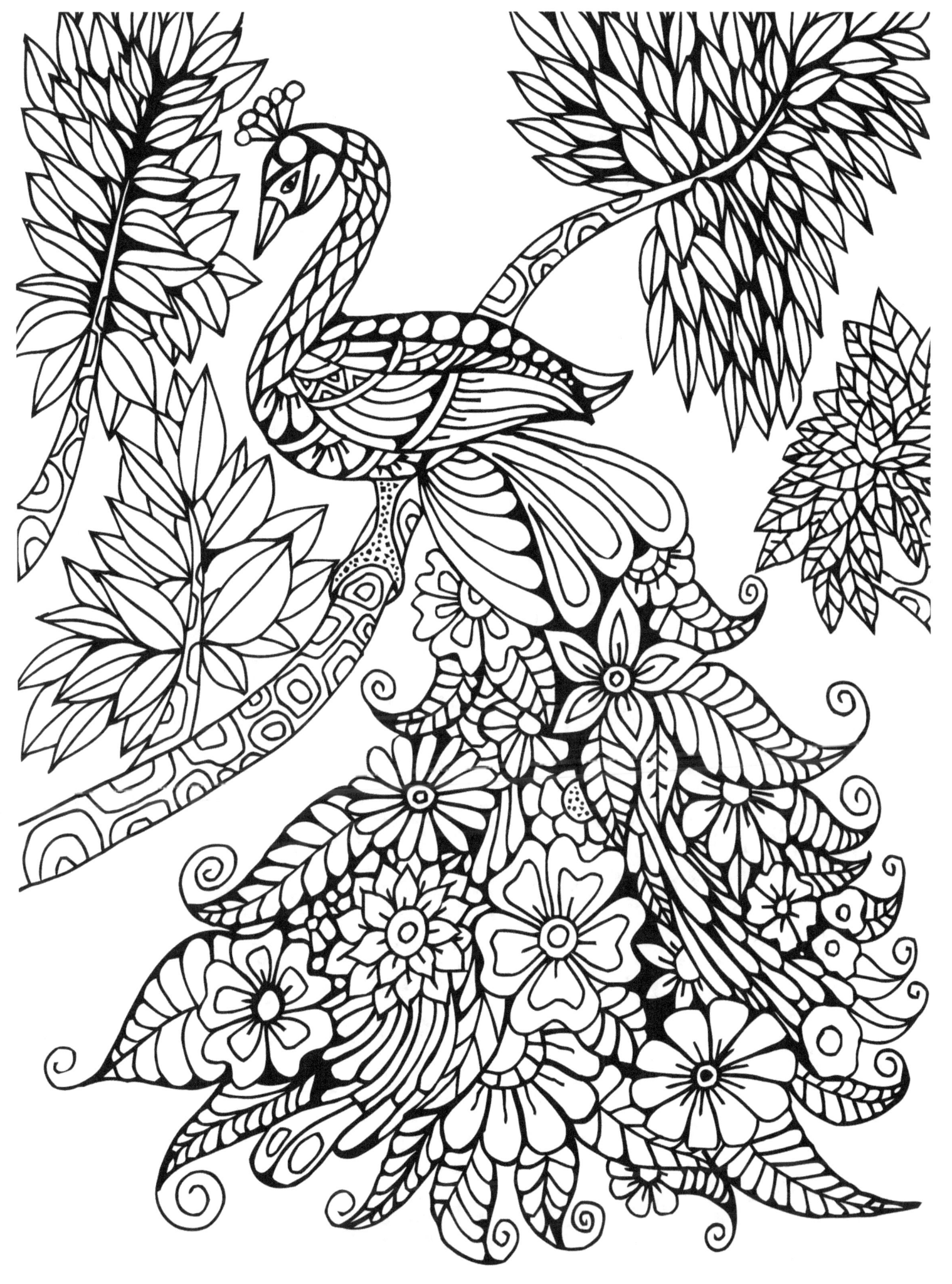

Left blank for your convenience

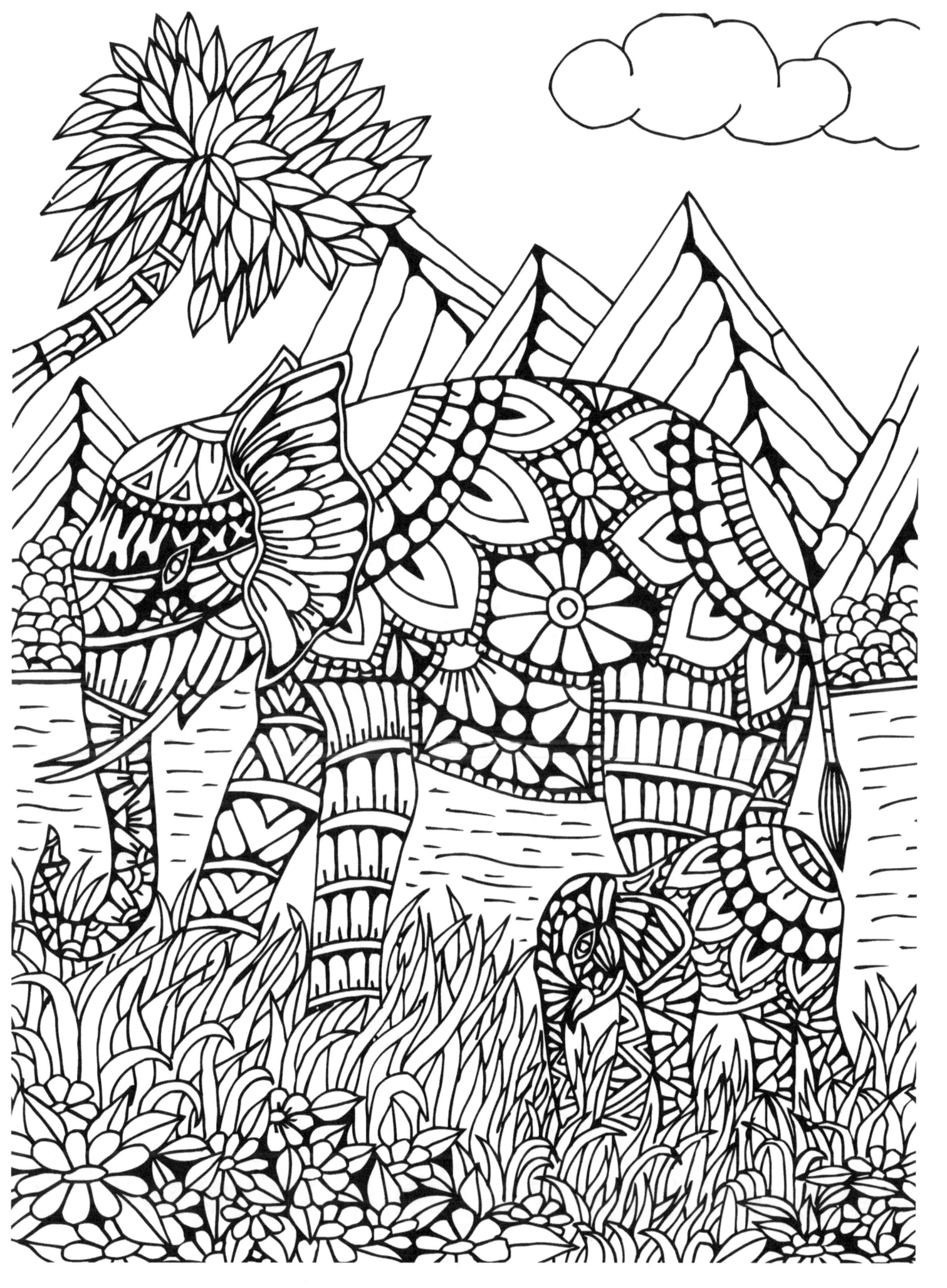

Left blank for your convenience

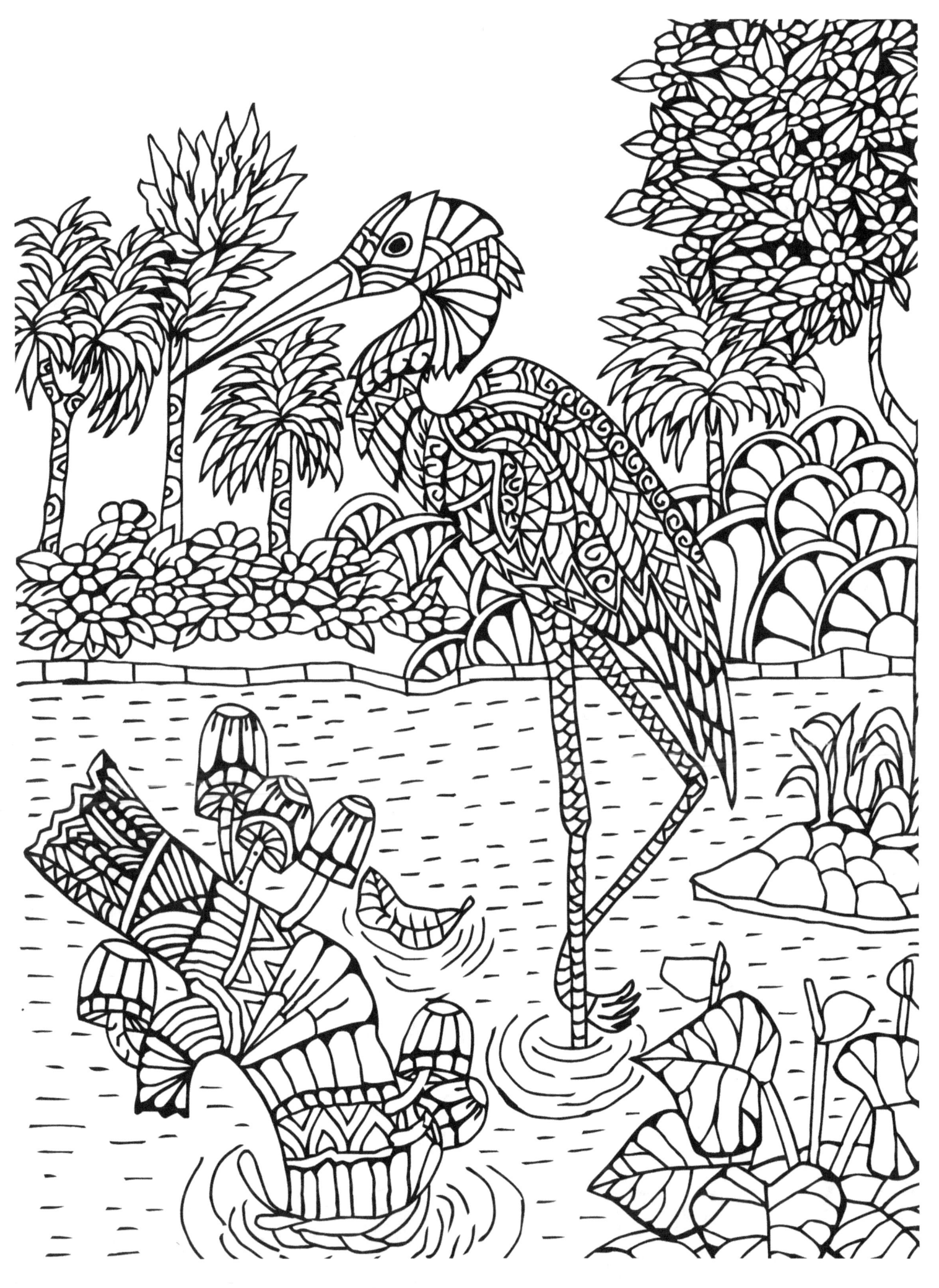

Left blank for your convenience

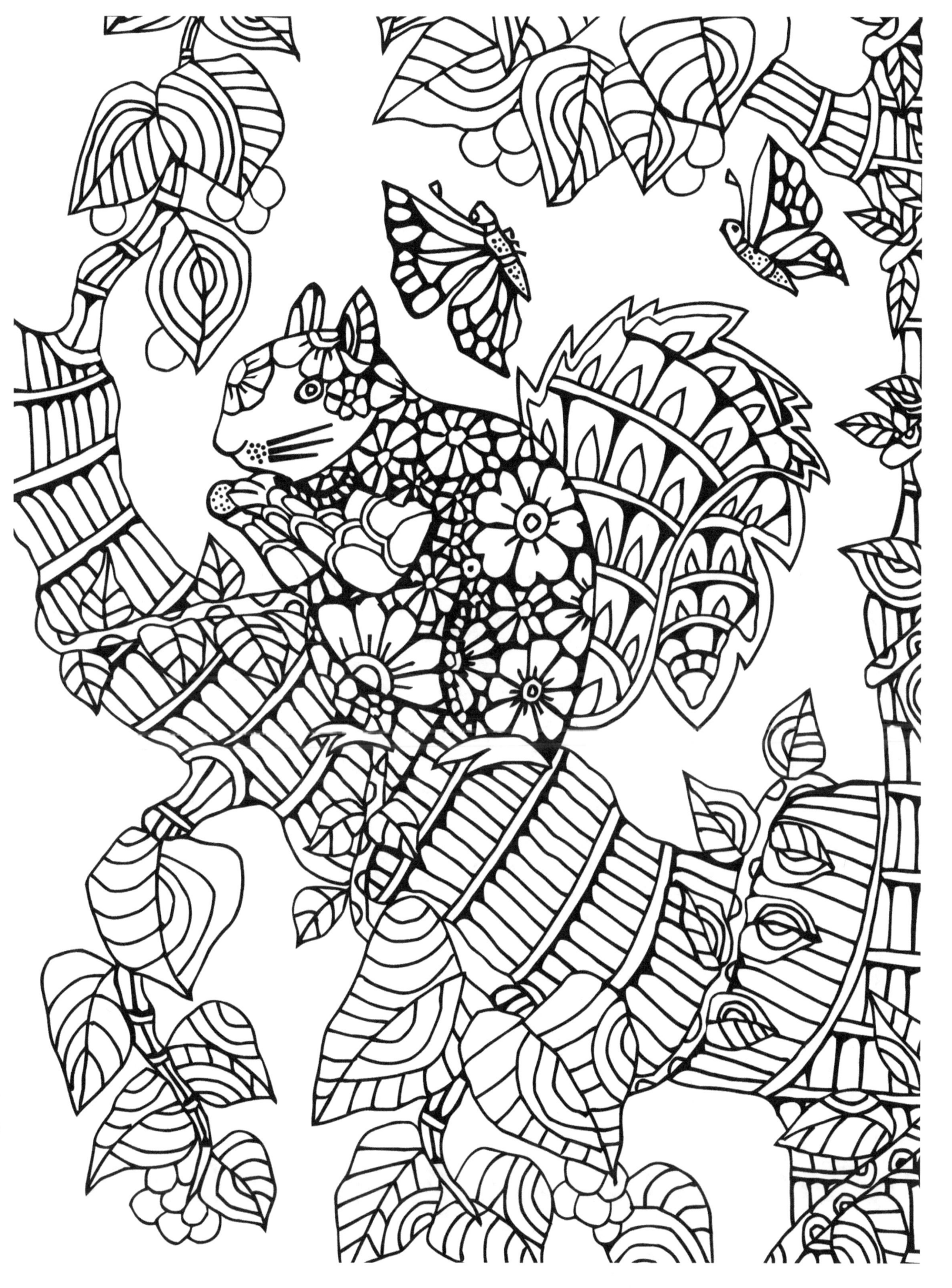

Left blank for your convenience

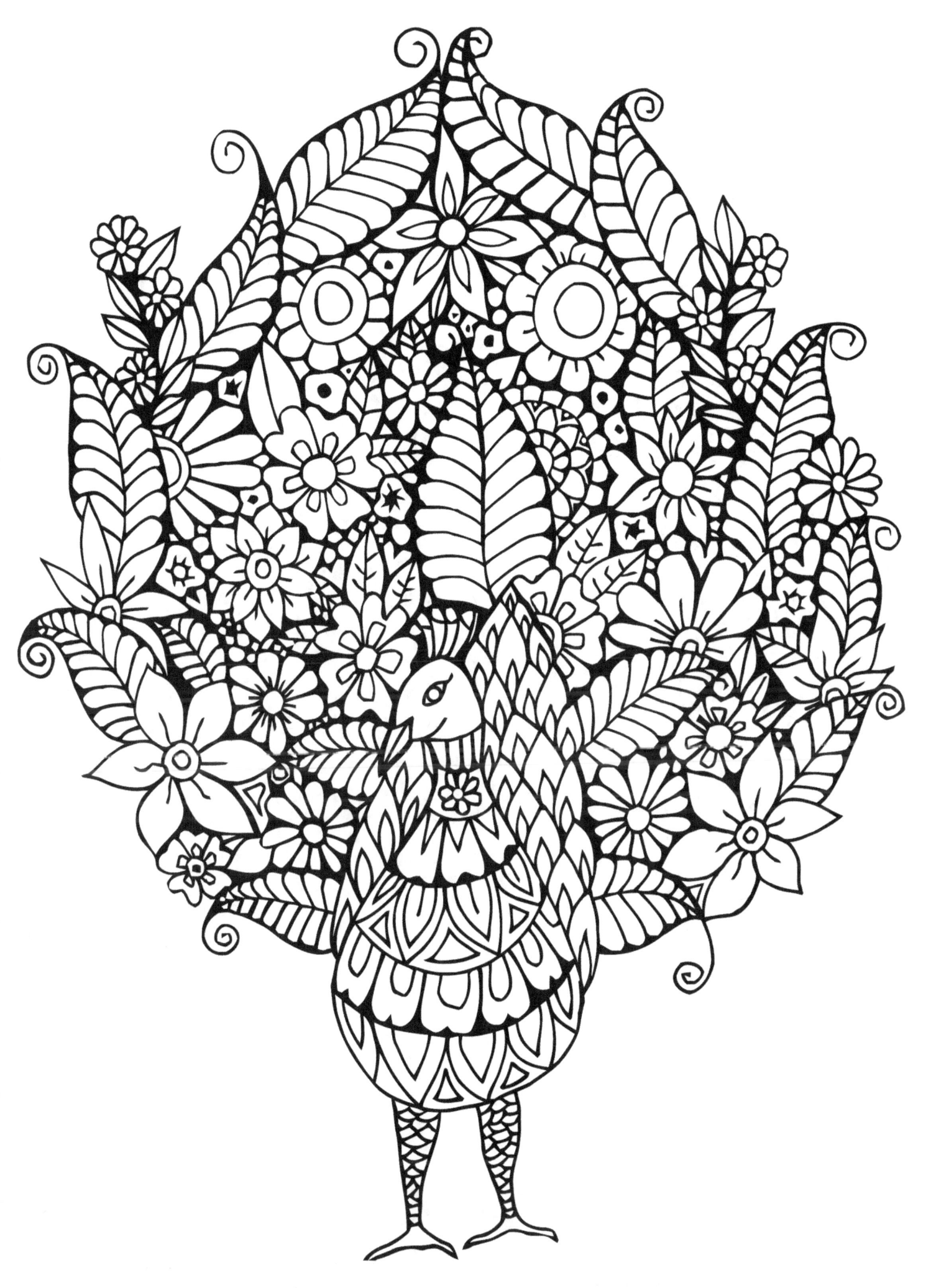

Left blank for your convenience

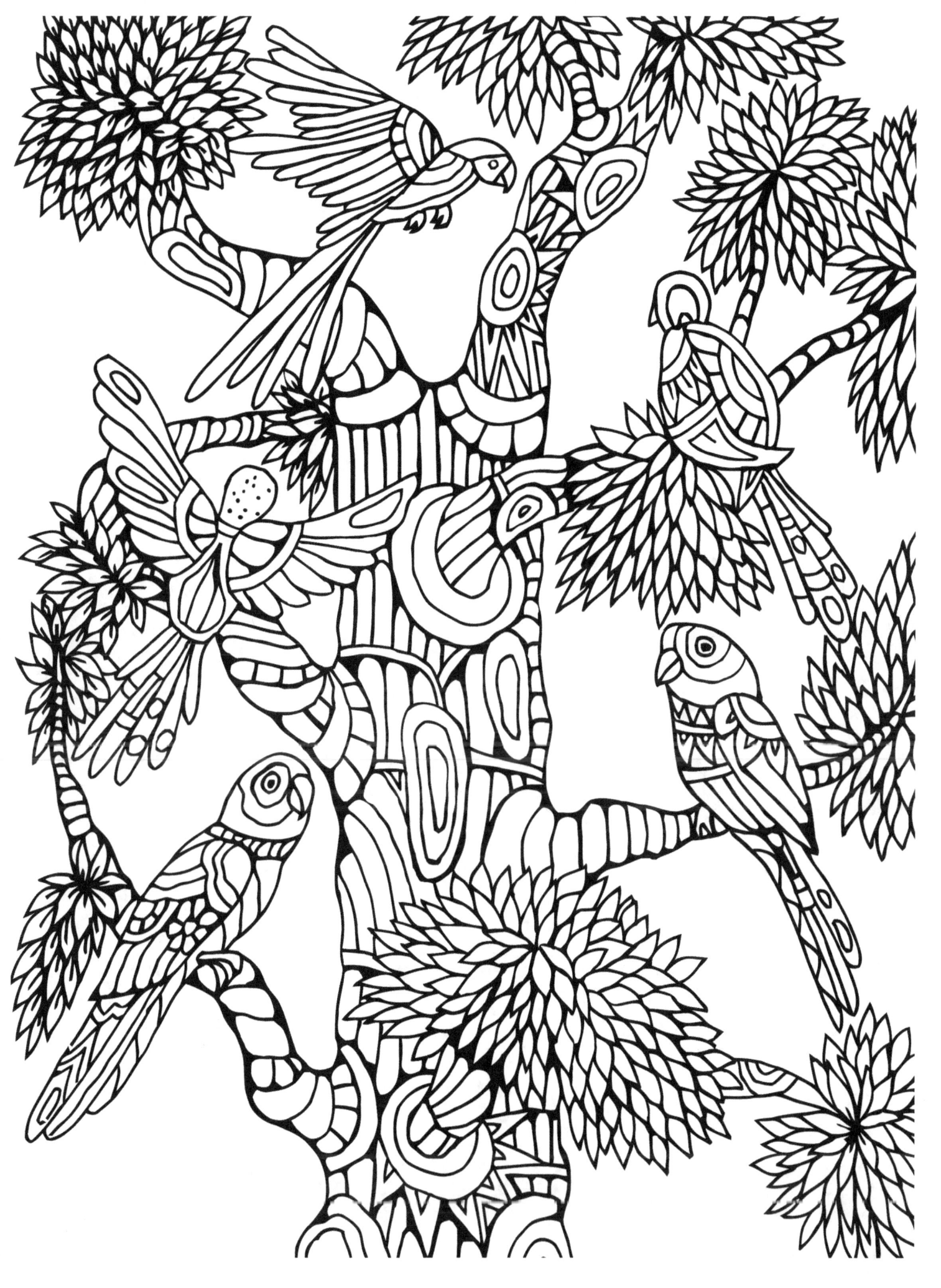

Left blank for your convenience

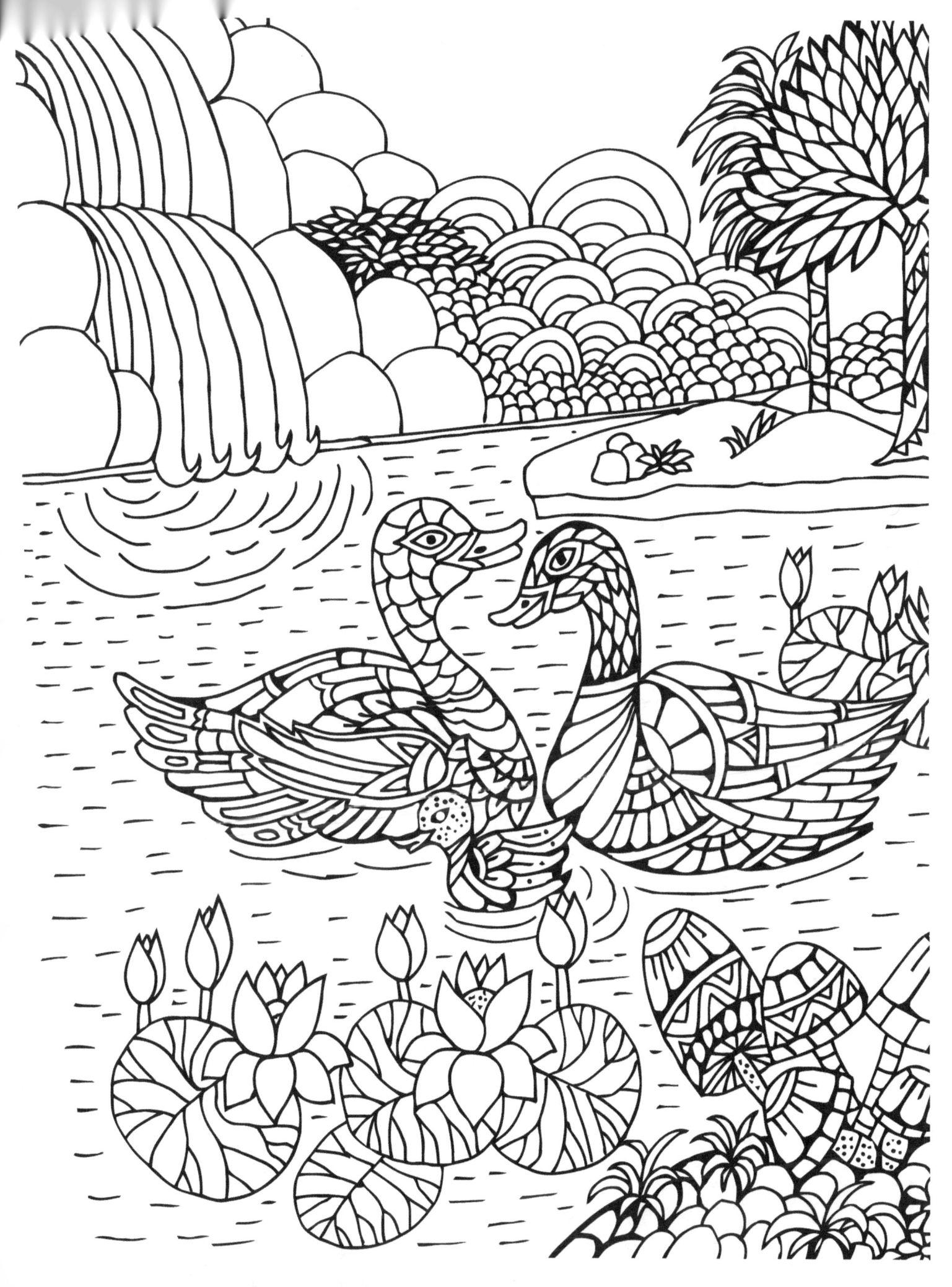

Left blank for your convenience

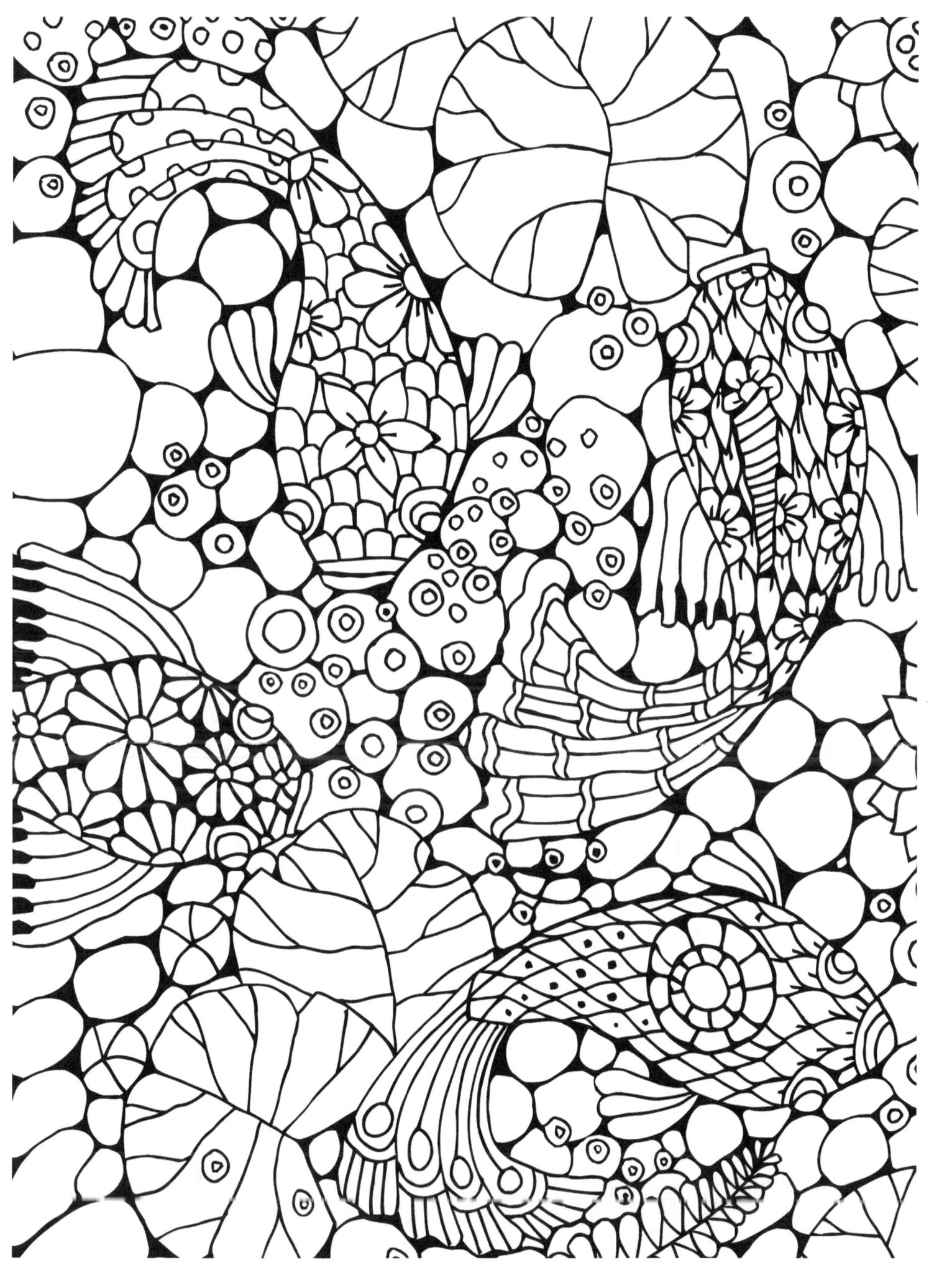

Left blank for your convenience

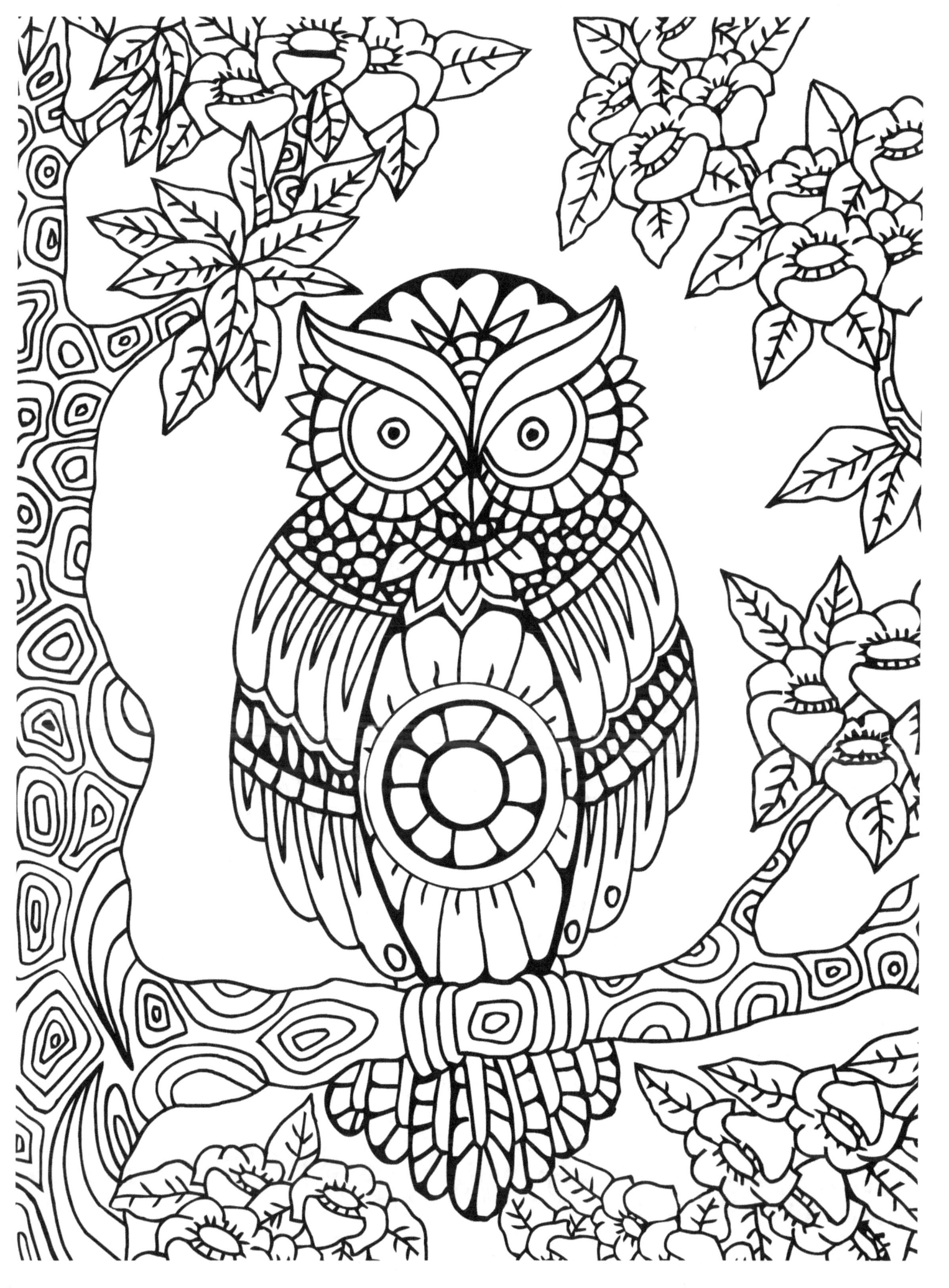

Left blank for your convenience

www.ingramcontent.com/pod-product-compliance
Lightning Source LLC
Chambersburg PA
CBHW081403280526
45788CB00009B/2967